The Pediatric Nurse's Survival Guide

The Pediatric Nurse's Survival Guide

SECOND EDITION

Lisa M. Rebeschi, RN, MSN, Doctoral Student
Assistant Professor
Southern Connecticut State University
New Haven, Connecticut

Mary Heiens Brown, PhD, RN, CPNP
Assistant Professor of Clinical Nursing
University of Texas at Houston
Health Science Center School of Nursing
Houston, Texas

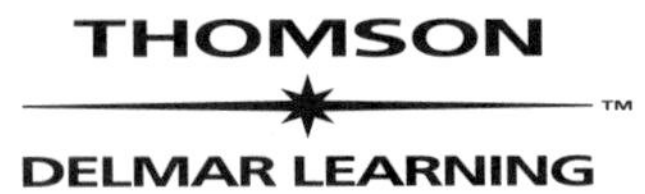

The Pediatric Nurse's Survival Guide
Second Edition
Lisa M. Rebeschi and Mary Heiens Brown

Business Unit Director:
William Brottmiller

Executive Editor:
Cathy L. Esperti

Acquisitions Editor:
Matthew Kane

Developmental Editor:
Marah E. Bellegarde

Executive Marketing Manager:
Dawn F. Gerrain

Channel Manager:
Jennifer McAvey

Editorial Assistant:
Shelley Esposito

Art and Design Coordinator:
Jay Purcell

Production Coordinator:
Anne Sherman

Project Editor:
David Buddle

Printed in the United States of America
1 2 3 4 5 XXX 06 05 04 02

For more information contact Delmar Learning, 5 Maxwell Drive, P.O. Box 8007, Clifton Park, NY 12065-8007

Or find us on the World Wide Web at http://www.delmar.com

Library of Congress Cataloging-in-Publication Data

Rebeschi, Lisa M.
The pediatric nurse's survival guide / written by Lisa M. Rebeschi and Mary H. Brown.—2nd ed.
p. cm.
Includes bibliographical references and index.
ISBN 0-7668-4952-X
1. Pediatric nursing—Handbooks, manuals, etc. I. Brown, Mary H., MSN II. Title.

RJ245 .R43 2002
610.73′62—dc21

2001054819

NOTICE TO THE READER

CONTENTS

PREFACE

The Pediatric Nurse's Survival Guide, second edition, is a concise pocket-size reference that includes applicable clinical information about laboratory values, common disorders, and medications commonly used with pediatric clients, as well as handy assessment information. *The Pediatric Nurse's Survival Guide* is designed to accompany any core pediatric textbook, or it can be used alone by practicing nurses who need a quick reference.

This second edition includes an expanded section on common health problems of the pediatric client. New additions include information on Kawasaki disease, streptococcal tonsillitis, eating disorders, depression, and post-traumatic stress disorder to name a few. The authors have included common nursing diagnoses found with each health problem. Nursing diagnoses have been updated to reflect *NANDA Nursing Diagnoses: Definitions and Classification 2001–2002.* New figures have been added, including the West nomogram, common injection sites, and stages of sexual development. The medication section has been updated to include the medications most commonly given to pediatric clients.

REVIEWERS

Vera V. Cull, RN, DSN
Birmingham School of Nursing
University of Alabama
Birmingham, Alabama

Judith W. Herrman, MS, RN
Department of Nursing
University of Delaware
Newark, Delaware

Linda Salmon, RN, BSN
Collins Career Center
Chesapeake, Ohio

Carolyn L. Walker, PhD, RN, CPON
School of Nursing
San Diego State University
San Diego, California

CHAPTER 1

COMMUNICATION

COMMUNICATING WITH CHILDREN AND FAMILIES

Communication skills are essential in providing quality nursing care. Nurses need to frequently assess perceptions to assess levels of understanding. Effective communication in the pediatric setting requires communication skills with both children and their caregiver(s).

Some of the basic principles to keep in mind are the following:

- Remember that privacy is an essential component
- Properly identify yourself, your role, and your purpose
- Ensure confidentiality, including maintaining safeguards for privacy of computerized patient data
- Be aware of environmental characteristics
- Begin communication with more general content before getting specific
- Communicate directly with the child even when accompanied by an adult
- Remember that adolescents may need to communicate in private without the presence of family members
- Use open-ended questions appropriately
- Encourage continued communication with nonverbal gestures such as nodding and eye contact
- Recognize and be respectful of cultural influences on communication
- Use interpreters as necessary
- Remember that silence is an appropriate communication technique
- Remember that active listening to both nonverbal and verbal cues is one of the most important components to effective communication
- Ensure mutual understanding by restating
- Avoid common communication blockers such as changing focus, falsely reassuring, interrupting, forming prejudged conclusions, and overloading with information
- Maintain eye-level position with child during communication
- Remember that transition objects such as stuffed animals may be useful when communicating with children

- Remember that writing, drawing, and playing are alternative communication approaches for older children
- Remember that honesty is of ultimate importance

CULTURALLY SENSITIVE APPROACHES

Nurses are continually challenged to meet the needs of a multicultural society as they provide care to diverse populations. Nurses recognize that culture plays an important role in the socialization of children and that cultural values are passed from one generation to the next by the family unit. A holistic view of children and families requires an understanding and respect of cultural influences.

Culture provides children and families with a sort of "blueprint" for living, thinking, behaving, and feeling. It guides the way in which individuals solve their problems and derive meaning from their lives.

To provide culturally sensitive care, nurses must evaluate their own feelings, prejudices, and beliefs. Nurses must make a conscious effort to recognize, appreciate, and respect differing views and beliefs of clients. Cultural sensitivity involves an awareness of both cultural similarities and differences.

The following are some general guidelines to follow in relation to cultural sensitivity:

- Avoid generalizations about ethnic groups because they may not apply
- Allow children and caregivers to select their own comfortable distance (also use this guide when touching clients)
- Observe family interactions to determine acceptable and appropriate gestures
- Observe cues regarding appropriate eye contact
- Always ask for clarification when uncertain
- Use positive tone of voice to convey genuine interest
- Encourage questions
- Learn basic words, gestures, and beliefs when family's culture and/or language is different from your own
- Use information written in family's native language
- Continually evaluate your own values and beliefs regarding other cultures

THE USE OF PLAY IN CHILDREN

Play is described as the "work" of children. It is crucial to maintain the activities of play with children who are hospitalized. Play serves several functions: sensorimotor development, intellectual development, socialization, moral development, creative outlets, avenue for self-awareness, and therapeutic value.

It is essential to consider safety concerns (e.g., size of item) when children are engaged in play. The following suggestions are play activities by age for children who are hospitalized:

Infants

- Colorful mobiles
- Music boxes
- Mirrors
- Infant swing
- "Pat-a-cake"
- Colored blocks
- Nested boxes or cups
- Large picture books

Toddlers

- Sing-along tapes
- Pull toys
- Riding toys (e.g., rocking horse)
- Wooden puzzles
- Finger paints
- Coloring with thick crayons
- Play dough
- Stuffed animals, dolls (check for safety)
- Television, videos, interactive computer games

Preschoolers

- Riding toys (e.g., tricycle)
- Puppets
- Drawing, coloring, cutting out pictures
- Scrapbooking
- Dolls, stuffed animals
- Dress up
- Jigsaw puzzles
- Books
- Musical toys
- Finger paints

School-aged Children

- Card playing
- Board games

- Drawing
- Movies, videos
- Interactive video games
- Play involving peer interaction

Adolescents

- Board games
- Audiotapes, CDs, radio
- Videos, movies
- Mental challenge games
- Craft activities

Therapeutic play may be used when the child is unable to completely verbalize his or her feelings. It is used to better understand the child's thoughts about hospitalization, procedures, fears, and concerns. Both verbal and nonverbal messages from the child are important. Drawing, painting, anatomically correct dolls, and direct play with medical equipment are often used. The following are some general guidelines for therapeutic play:

- Allow as much choice as possible for children to select articles to play with
- Allow the child to play with actual medical materials that he or she will be confronted with (e.g., stethoscope, nasogastric [NG] tube, tympanic thermometer)
- Use therapeutic communication techniques
- Ask the child to describe his or her drawings
- Always supervise therapeutic play
- Consult with child life therapists if available

CHAPTER 2

ASSESSMENT

PHYSICAL ASSESSMENT

General Guidelines

The physical assessment of a pediatric client must be performed as opportunities present. Therefore, be prepared with all equipment, including stethoscope, tape measure, penlight, and tongue blade, when entering a client's room. The assessment should begin immediately. The client's skin color, position, and gait (if the child is observed walking) should be noted, as well as the caregiver's response and caregiver-child interaction. If an infant is sleeping, it is a good time to listen to his or her heart sounds. Rapport can be established with the caregiver and child by talking first with the caregiver and then with the child. If the nurse has to leave the room to retrieve forgotten equipment, rapport with the child will have to be reestablished.

The nurse can use play therapy as necessary to accomplish his or her assessment of the child. Listening to the caregiver's or a stuffed toy's heart and lungs can show children, especially toddlers, that it does not hurt. The nurse can then attempt to obtain resting heart rate, heart sounds, respirations, and breath sounds. The child also can be allowed to assist with the assessment as he or she is able. Preschoolers and older children like to listen to their own heart sounds. This is a valuable opportunity to teach a child about the body and how to keep it healthy, as well as to validate the child's normalcy.

Invasive procedures and painful areas or procedures should be saved until the end of the assessment. What constitutes invasive varies with age groups. For example, examining ears, mouth, and nose is invasive to toddlers. Genitourinary system and abdominal procedures are invasive to school-aged children and adolescents. If the child refuses to cooperate, the nurse must use a firm approach and perform the examination as quickly as possible. Regardless of the order in which the assessment is performed, it must be charted in a logical head-to-toe format.

General Appearance

Note overall impression of the child. For example, is the child small, obese, well nourished, awake, alert, cooperative, developmentally appropriate for age, lethargic, or distressed? What is the client's state of consciousness?

Skin

Inspect and palpate the skin for color. (Remember that room color, gown color, and lighting affect observation. Evaluate for jaundice in natural lighting of a window; cyanosis blanches momentarily, bruises do not.) Also note pigmentation, temperature, texture, moisture, and turgor.

Note and describe all lesions for the following:

Location—exactly where on body
Pattern—clustered, confluent, evanescent, linear
Size—measured in centimeters
Color—red, pink, brown, white, hyperpigmented, or hypopigmented
Elevation—raised (papular), flat (macular), fluid filled (vesicular)
Blanching—do they pale when pressure is applied?

Hair

Note color, texture, distribution, quality, and loss. Look in hair behind the ears for nits.

Nails

Note color, cyanosis, shape, and condition of nails. Clubbing is determined by checking nail angle. The normal angle is 160 degrees. An angle of 180 degrees or larger is seen in clubbing caused by hypoxia.

Head

Inspect and palpate the child's head, feeling for bogginess, sutures, and fontanels. Posterior fontanel normally closes from birth to 2 months and is usually 1 to 2 cm in size. Anterior fontanel normally closes between 9 and 18 months but should be closed by 2 years. Measure anterior fontanel in two dimensions; usually is 4 to 5 cm by 3 to 4 cm, but should be at least 1 cm by 1 cm. Normally, the fontanels should feel flat. In states of dehydration, fontanels may be sunken. In states of increased intracranial pressure, fontanels may be bulging. Measure frontal occipital circumference (FOC) until the child is 36 months old or if its size is important to the child's condition after 2 years of age. Always plot FOC and note size, shape, and symmetry of the head. Palpate the scalp for tenderness and lesions.

Neck

Inspect the neck for swelling, webbing, nuchal fold, and vein distension. Palpate for swelling, carotid pulse, trachea, and thyroid.

Ears

Inspect the ears for shape, color, symmetry, helix formation, and position. The top of the ear should go through an imaginary line from the inner canthus to the outer canthus to the occiput. Palpate for firmness and pain and observe for and describe any discharge from the ear canal. Assess for gross hearing. Infants less than 4 months of age startle to sound. Older infants turn to localize the sound of jingling keys and other objects. Use the whisper test with verbal and cooperative children.

Eyes

Inspect the eyes for position, alignment, lid closure, inner canthal distance (average = 2.5 cm), epicanthal folds, and slant of fissure. Note dark circles under the eyes (usually present in children with allergies).

- Brows—note separateness, nits
- Lashes—note if they curve into eye
- Lids—note color, swelling, lesions, discharge
- Conjunctiva
  - Palpebral (should be pink)—note redness, pallor
  - Sclera and bulbar—note injection, redness, color (should be white; yellow in jaundice, blue in osteogenesis imperfecta)
- Pupils—note shape, size, and briskness of reaction to light by constricting directly and consensually and accommodation for near and far vision
- Iris—note color, roundness, any clefts or defects
- Extraocular movements (EOMs)
  - Six cardinal fields of gaze—Hold child's chin and have him or her follow your finger, moving in the shape of an H, with his or her eyes to note asymmetric eye movement or to elicit nystagmus; a few beats of nystagmus in the far lateral gaze are normal.
  - Corneal light reflex—Hold light 15 inches from bridge of nose and shine on bridge. It should reflect in the same place in each eye in normally aligned eyes.
  - Cover–uncover test—Check for movement when one eye is covered and the other is gazing at a distant object. Remove cover and note movement of covered eye. Repeat using a near object.
- Gross vision—Newborns blink and hyperextend their necks to light. Infants who can see fix on and follow objects. Grossly assess older

children's vision by having them describe what they see on the wall or out the window.

Face

Note color, symmetrical movement, expression, skin folds, and swelling of the face.

Nose

Inspect the nose for color of skin, any nasal crease, nasal mucosa, any discharge and its color, and patency. Flaring of nares may be a sign of respiratory distress. Assess turbinates by shining a light into the nares while pushing up gently on the tip of the nose (red and swollen indicates possible upper respiratory infection; pale and boggy indicates possible allergic rhinitis). Infants are obligate nose breathers until approximately 3 months of age. Palpate sinuses for tenderness. Frontal sinuses are not developed completely until approximately 8 years of age.

Mouth

Inspect all areas of the mouth. Note number and condition of teeth. To calculate the expected number of teeth in infants, subtract 6 from the infant's age in months (e.g., 12 months−6=6 teeth). Observe tonsils for swelling (grade 1+ indicates mild swelling; grade 4+ indicates touching, or "kissing," tonsils), color (should be same color as buccal mucosa), and discharge. Examine the hard and soft palate for color, patency, and lesions. The uvula should rise symmetrically; a bifid uvula could indicate a submucosal cleft. Note tongue shape, size, color, movement and inspect for any lesions (most common lesions are white and are thrush). Note breath odor.

Thorax and Lungs

Inspect for symmetry, movement, color, retractions, breast development, and type and effort of breathing. Breathing is predominately abdominal until age 7 years. Note nasal flaring and use of accessory muscles. Retractions usually start subcostal and substernal, then progress to suprasternal and supraclavicular, and lastly intercostal, indicating severe distress. Palpate for tactile fremitus (increased in congestion and consolidation). Percuss for resonance (sound becomes dull with fluid or masses). Auscultate side to side for symmetry of sound. Infants breathe deeper when they cry; toddlers and preschoolers can breathe deeper when they blow bubbles or try to "blow out the light" of your pen light. Assess all fields. Listen to the back to assess the lower lobes in children younger than 8 years of age. Auscultate in the axillae to best hear crackles in children with suspected pneumonia. Normal sounds are vesicular or bronchovesicular. Infants' breath sounds are louder and more bronchial because they have thin chest walls.

Describe adventitious sounds as follows:

- Rhonchi—a continuous, low-pitched sound with a snoring quality
- Crackles—intermittent, brief, repetitive sounds caused by small collapsed airways popping open
  - Fine crackles—soft, high-pitched and brief
  - Coarse crackles—louder, lower-pitched and slightly longer than fine crackles
- Wheezes—musical, more continuous sounds produced by rapid movement of air through narrowed passages
  - Usual progression of wheezing starts with expiratory wheezes only, then inspiratory wheezes with decreased expiratory wheezes, then inspiratory wheezes only (airways are collapsing on expiration), and finally, no sounds because there is little air movement.
- Stridor—inspiratory wheeze heard louder in neck than in chest, usually right over trachea

Infants with upper airway congestion can have sounds transmitted to lungs because they are obligate nose breathers. Listen to their lungs when they are crying and breathing through their mouths to decrease the amount of transmitted noise and better assess their breath sounds.

Cardiovascular System

Inspect for point of maximum impulse (PMI), cyanosis, mottling, edema, respiratory distress, clubbing, activity intolerance, and tiring with feeds. Palpate PMI and brachial, radial, femoral, and pedal pulses.

Auscultate the following areas with bell and diaphragm of the stethoscope:

Aortic area	Right second intercostal space (ICS) at right sternal border (SB)
Pulmonic area	Left second ICS at left SB
Erb's point	Left third ICS at left SB
Tricuspid	Left fifth ICS at left SB
Mitral	Left fifth ICS at left midclavicular line

S_1 correlates with the carotid pulse and is best heard at the apex of the heart. S_2 is best heard in the aortic and pulmonic areas (base of heart). Quality of sound should be crisp and clear. Heart rate should be normal for age and condition and synchronous with the radial pulse. Rhythm should be regular or may slow and speed up with respirations in young infants.

Auscultate with the child in two positions if possible. Auscultate for muffled or additional sounds and note where these are best heard.

Murmurs should be assessed for the following:

- Location—where heard best on the chest wall
- Timing in cardiac cycle—continuous, systolic, or diastolic
- Grade—I/VI to VI/VI
  - I/VI—very faint, have to really tune in
  - II/VI—quiet, but can hear soon after placing stethoscope
  - III/VI—moderately loud
  - IV/VI—loud
  - V/VI—very loud, may be heard with stethoscope partially off chest
  - VI/VI—can hear without stethoscope
- Pitch—high (best heard with the diaphragm), medium, or low (best heard with the bell)
- Quality—harsh, blowing, machinery-like, musical
- Radiation—does it radiate, and if so where (listen to back, axillae, and above clavicles)

Abdomen

Inspect the abdomen for pulsation, contour, symmetry, peristaltic waves, masses, and normal skin color. Auscultate before palpating so that normal bowel sounds are not disturbed. Listen in all four quadrants for a full minute. Normal sounds should be heard every 10 to 30 seconds; should hear 4 to 5 sounds per minute. Less than 4 per minute indicates decreased bowel sounds. Listen for a full 5 minutes before concluding that they are absent.

Percuss for dullness over the client's liver and full bladder. The rest of the abdomen should percuss tympani. Palpate using light pressure first. Have the child bend the knees up while lying on his or her back to relax the abdomen. Use the child's hands under your hands if the child is very ticklish or tense. With deep palpation, support the child from the back, then palpate. Start in lower quadrants and move upward to detect an enlarged liver or spleen. Note areas of tenderness, pain, or any masses.

Anus

Inspect the skin and perineum for excoriation, bruising, discoloration, or tears.

Genitourinary System

- Female genitalia—Note redness, excoriation, discharge and odor.
- Male genitalia—Note if circumcised or uncircumcised. (If uncircumcised, see if foreskin is retractable.) Note position of meatus. Close off

the canals and feel for the testes or any masses in the scrotal sac. If you feel a mass other than the testes, transilluminate for fluid. Hydroceles are fluid in the scrotal sac and will transilluminate light. Hernias are loops of bowel and will not transilluminate.

Lymphatic System

Palpate the lymphatic system throughout the examination with the pads of the fingers. Nodes should be firm, small (1 cm or less), freely moveable, and nontender. Palpate preauricular, postauricular, anterior and posterior cervical chains, supraclavicular and subclavicular, axillary, and inguinal lymph nodes.

Musculoskeletal System

Incorporate assessment of the musculoskeletal system into rest of the examination. Observe walking, sitting, turning, and range of motion in all joints. Observe spinal curvature and mobility. Exaggerated lumbar curve is normal in toddlers. Note sacral dimples or tufts of hair at the base of the spinal column. Note symmetry and movement of the extremities.

Test muscle strength. Strength is graded on a 0 to 5 scale. Normal muscle strength is grade 5.

0—no contraction noted
1—barely a trace of contraction
2—active movement without gravity
3—active movement against gravity
4—active movement against gravity and resistance
5—active movement against full resistance without tiring

Note size, color, temperature, and mobility of joints. Examine palmar creases. A single crease is a *simian crease* and can be associated with Down syndrome. Note extra digits and deformities. Thumb deformities may be associated with heart defects.

Note stance and gait. Bowed legs (genu varum) are normal in toddlers until approximately age 2 years. Knock-knees (genu valgum) are normal from 2 until approximately 6 to 10 years. Note foot deformities. Stroke the side of the foot to see if it returns to a neutral position. Check for dislocatable hips using Barlow's test and Ortolani's maneuver. Also look for uneven skin folds.

Nervous System

Observe grossly for speech and ability to follow directions in an older child. In an infant, observe activity and tone. In ambulatory patients, observe gait and balance.

Check deep tendon reflexes. These are graded from 0 to 4+.

4+—very brisk, hyperactive
3+—brisker than average
2+—normal
1+—decreased
0—absent

Use a percussion hammer or the side of the stethoscope diaphragm to elicit the following responses:

Deep Tendon Reflex	Procedure	Response
Biceps	Hit antecubital space	Forearm flexes
Triceps	Bend arm at elbow, hit triceps tendon above elbow	Forearm extends
Patellar	Strike patellar tendon	Lower leg extends
Achilles	Hold foot lightly, hit Achilles tendon	Foot flexes downward
Cranial nerves	Most are integrated into routine examination and are not specifically tested.	

INFANT REFLEXES

Reflex	Age	Assessment
Babinski	Birth to 2 yr	Stroke bottom of foot; toes fan
Galant	Birth to 4–8 wk	Stroke infant's side; hips swing to that side
Moro	Birth to 3–4 mo	Arms extend, fingers fan (if asymmetrical, brachial plexus injury should be suspected); if Moro persists beyond 6 mo, brain damage should be suspected
Palmar grasp	Birith to 4 mo	Put your finger in infant's palm from ulnar side; infant closes fingers around your finger
Rooting	Birth to 4 mo (up to 12 mo during sleep)	Stroke infant's cheek and corner of mouth; infant's head turns in that direction
Sucking	Birth to 4 mo (7 mo during sleep)	Infant has reflexive sucking to stimuli

Neurovascular System

Assess the neurovascular system very closely in children with intravenous (IV) lines in extremities, and those in casts, restraints, and in traction. Note color and size of extremity and compare with unaffected extremity. Check pulses bilaterally for equality of strength. Check capillary refill time by pinching a toe or finger and noting the time it takes for the color to return. They should have brisk, immediate blood return. Both congestive heart failure and dehydration can increase capillary refill time. Assess for any alterations in sensation or increased pain.

NEONATAL VARIANCES IN ASSESSMENT

General

Note overall impression, (e.g., alert, awake, sleepy, responsive). Note cry intensity and pitch. High-pitched cry is associated with increased intracranial pressure.

Skin

- Color (assess before disturbing)
  - Plethora—Ruddy, red color associated with a high hematocrit
  - Acrocyanosis—Cyanosis of the hands and feet; normal in first few days
  - Jaundice—Yellow color; common after first 24 hr; assess in natural light
  - Bruising—Common with difficult deliveries; facial bruising common in face presentations and in infants with nuchal cords (cord around the neck)
  - Petechiae—Normal on face and upper trunk in rapid deliveries
  - Cyanosis—Assess for cause (cyanosis will blanch, bruises will not)
- Pustular melanosis—Small pustules at birth that reveal freckles when burst; common finding in infants with dark skin; persists approximately 3 to 4 months
- Erythema toxicum neonaterum—“Normal newborn rash”; evanescent rash characterized by small yellow pustules on an erythematous base; most common in infants with fair skin; usually appears after first 24 hr and lasts up to 2 weeks
- Peeling skin—Associated with postmaturity
- Milia—Small white dots usually present on nose and/or chin; caused by blocked sweat glands; resolve by 2 to 4 months
- Nevus flammeus—“Stork Bites,” also called salmon patches; most commonly on the nape of the neck and eyelids; turn bright red when infant cries; usually fade over the first year
- Mongolian spots—Normal hyperpigmented areas most commonly seen in infants with dark skin; usually on sacral area, but can be anywhere; may be purple, blue, green, or brown

Hair

Note whorls, abnormal coloring or distribution of hair. Color may change. Infants lose initial hair, which is replaced with permanent hair during the first 6 months. Some lose it gradually, and some all at once. In fact, bald spots from rubbing the head on the mattress are common.

Nails

Infants' nails may be meconium stained. The longer the nails, the more mature the infant.

Head

Note anterior and posterior fontanels. They may appear larger than normal because of open sagittal or frontal sutures. This is not of concern if FOC is normal. Sutures may override as a result of molding to fit in the birth canal. Sutures should be flat by 6 months. Measure and plot FOC to determine microcephaly or hydrocephaly. Note electrode marks and observe them daily for infection.

Caput succedaneum—Diffuse swelling, usually over occiput, that crosses suture lines and is usually resolved in the first few days

Cephalohematoma—Distinct swelling that does not cross suture lines; caused by bleeding into the periosteum; calcifies then absorbs; persists about 3–4 months

Craniotabes—A "ping-pong ball" effect of the bone usually caused by thin cranial bones; normal near the sutures, abnormal where the bones should be thick; can be indicative of hydrocephaly or syphilis

Neck

The neck is usually short. Note webbing (common in Turner's syndrome) and nuchal folds (normal variation in large infants or associated with other findings in Down syndrome).

Ears

Note position of ears. Low set ears are associated with renal abnormalities and hearing loss. A rolled or flat helix usually is a result of intrauterine position. Assess for gross hearing. Newborns should blink to loud noises (acoustical blink reflex). Note preauricular pits and tags. Pits usually are not significant, but large tags can be associated with hearing problems.

Eyes

Note position and alignment of the eyes. Note red reflex bilaterally. Cloudy red reflex is associated with congenital cataracts. White reflexes are associated with retinoblastoma. Red reflexes in infants with dark skin are not bright red, but rather a more pinkish-gray as a result of pigment. Lids may be puffy because of chemical conjunctivitis caused by prophylactic drops given at birth. Short palpebral fissures may be associated with fetal alcohol syndrome.

Face

The infant's face may be asymmetrical because of intrauterine position. Assess for symmetry of movement, especially if forceps were used during delivery. Note abnormal facial features.

Nose

The infant's nose may be asymmetrical because of intrauterine position. Assess for patency. Infants are obligate nose breathers until 3 months of age.

Mouth

Assess the palate and suck and gag reflexes. Note any natal teeth. A large tongue may be associated with hypothyroidism and Down syndrome. Note any ankyloglossia (tongue-tie); this may interfere with successful breastfeeding if the tongue is too tightly anchored to the floor of the mouth.

Thorax and Lungs

Breast engorgement with or without milky discharge is normal in both sexes and is associated with maternal hormones. This resolves without intervention but may persist for up to 6 months, or longer in breastfed infants. Supranummary or extra nipples are common. These will not develop further.

A newborn's xiphoid process curves upward and normally is very prominent. Breath sounds should be equal bilaterally and usually sound louder because of a thin chest wall. Note tachypnea (respiratory rate >60), grunting, flaring, and retractions.

Cardiovascular System

Assess an infant's cardiovascular system as with an older child. Grades II to III/VI murmurs are common at the upper left sternal border (LSB); continuous sound usually indicates a patent ductus arteriosus. Systolic murmurs at the upper LSB usually are transient and benign. Murmurs at the mid-LSB or lower LSB bear watching. Compare brachial and femoral pulses. If femoral pulses are diminished or absent, check and compare blood pressures from the four extremities.

Abdomen

The umbilical cord should have three vessels (two arteries and one vein). The cord should be treated with alcohol and should dry and fall off within the first 3 weeks. Umbilical hernias are present in 90% of newborns and are normal. Note the size of any defects in the abdominal wall. If the rectus muscle is not fused at birth, the infant has diastasis recti. This is a normal finding and usually closes by itself during the first year. The liver normally is palpated at the costal margin or down 2 cm; in preterm infants it should not be palpated down more than half way to the umbilicus. The spleen normally is not palpated.

Anus

Check patency of the anus.

Genitourinary System

Male—Foreskin normally tight and meatus not visualized; testes may be retractile or in the canals

Female—Hypertrophied hymen or hymenal tag caused by maternal hormones is common and recedes as maternal hormonal influence fades; may have clear vaginal discharge that turns white, then bloody like a menstrual period before it goes away; once resolved, it should not return; prominent labial minora is normal in preterm infants

Lymphatic System

Nodes usually are not palpable.

Musculoskeletal System

Feel for crepitus over the clavicles. Fractures are common in large infants. With an asymmetrical Moro reflex, suspect brachial plexus injury. Feel all long bones for crepitus. Note tone. "Floppy" babies with significantly decreased tone need to be assessed further for hypoglycemia, perinatal drug exposure, sepsis, and/or chromosomal abnormalities. Extra digits originating at the second knuckle of the fifth digit of the hand are very common in African-American infants.

Nervous System

Check normal infant reflexes. Infants who are jittery need to be assessed for hypoglycemia and perinatal drug exposure.

al Signs

MAL TEMPERATURES IN CHILDREN

	Temperature (in degrees)	
	Fahrenheit	Celsius
3 mo	99.4	37.5
6 mo	99.5	37.5
1 yr	99.7	37.7
3 yr	99.0	37.2
5 yr	98.6	37.0
7 yr	98.3	36.8
9 yr	98.1	36.7
11 yr	98.0	36.7
13 yr	97.8	36.6

$F=(C \times 9/5) + 32$

$C=(F - 32) \times 5/9$

NORMAL HEART RATES IN CHILDREN

Age	Awake at rest (bpm)	Asleep (bpm)	Exercise/Fever (bpm)
Newborn	100–180	80–160	up to 220
1 wk to 3 mo	100–220	80–200	up to 220
3 mo to 2 yr	80–150	70–120	up to 200
2 to 10 yr	70–110	60–90	up to 200
10 yr to adult	55–90	50–90	up to 200

bpm, beats per minute.

Adapted from Potts, N. L., & Mandleco, B. L. (2002). *Pediatric nursing: Caring for children and their families*. Albany, NY: Delmar.

GRADING OF PULSES

Grade	Description
0	Not palpable
+1	Difficult to palpate; thready; weak; can be easily obliterated with pressure
+2	Difficult to palpate; may be obliterated with pressure
+3	Easy to palpate; not easily obliterated
+4	Strong; bounding; not obliterated with pressure

NORMAL RESPIRATORY RATES FOR CHILDREN

Age	Rate (breaths per minute)
Newborn	35
1–11 mo	30
2 yr	25
4 yr	23
6 yr	21
8 yr	20
10–12 yr	19
14 yr	18
16 yr	17
18 yr	16–18

Adapted from Potts, N. L., & Mandleco, B. L. (2002). *Pediatric nursing: Caring for children and their families*. Albany, NY: Delmar.

ASSESSMENT OF NORMAL BREATH SOUNDS

Classification	Description
Vesicular	Heard over entire lung surface, except upper intrascapular area and below manubrium
Bronchovesicular	Heard over manubrium and in upper intrascapular areas where trachea and bronchi bifurcate; inspirations are louder and higher in pitch than in vesicular breathing
Bronchial	Heard only near suprasternal notch over trachea; inspiratory phase is short and expiratory phase is long

NORMAL BLOOD PRESSURE RATES IN CHILDREN (BASED ON 50TH PERCENTILE)

	Females		Males	
Age	**Systolic**	**Diastolic**	**Systolic**	**Diastolic**
1 day	65	55	73	55
3 days	72	55	74	55
7 days	78	54	76	54
1 mo	84	52	86	52
2 mo	87	51	91	50
3 mo	90	51	91	50
4 mo	90	52	91	50
5 mo	91	52	91	52
6 mo	91	53	90	53
7 mo	91	53	90	54
8 mo	91	53	90	55
9 mo	91	54	90	55

10 mo	91	54	90	56
11 mo	91	54	90	56
1 yr	91	54	90	56
2 yr	90	56	91	56
3 yr	91	56	92	55
4 yr	92	56	93	56
5 yr	94	56	95	56
6 yr	96	57	96	57
7 yr	97	58	97	58
8 yr	99	59	99	60
9 yr	100	61	101	61
10 yr	102	62	102	62
11 yr	105	64	105	63
12 yr	107	66	107	64
13 yr	109	64	109	63
14 yr	110	67	112	64
15 yr	111	67	114	65
16 yr	112	67	117	67
17 yr	112	66	119	69
18 yr	112	66	121	70

Adapted from Potts, N. L., & Mandleco, B. L. (2002). *Pediatric nursing: Caring for children and their families*. Albany, NY: Delmar.

Growth Measurements

One of the most important areas in assessing children is the measurement of physical growth. The pediatric nurse should measure weight, height/length, head circumference, skinfold thickness, and arm circumference. Measurements are plotted on growth charts to determine percentiles to compare an individual child's measurements with that of the general population.

The National Center for Health Statistics (NCHS) has developed growth charts according to age. There is one growth chart to be used for children from birth to 36 months of age. In this age group, the weight by age, recumbent length by age, weight for length, and head circumference by age are plotted. There is another growth chart to be used for children ages 2 to 18 years. In this age group, weight by age and stature by age are plotted (see charts on pages 22–25).

The NCHS uses the 5th and 95th percentiles as the parameters for determining if children fall outside of the normal limits for growth. Those below the 5th percentile are considered underweight and/or small in stature and those above the 95th percentile are considered overweight and/or large in stature. Children whose measurements fall below or above the 95th percentile should be followed more closely, especially when genetic factors are not involved.

Recumbent length should be measured when the birth to 36-month growth chart is being used. The nurse should fully extend the infant's or child's body. The child should be placed on a papered surface and the nurse should mark the measurements at the top of the head and the heel of the foot. The child is then removed from the surface and the surface is measured with a tape measure.

Height is measured when using the 2- to 18-year growth chart. Height refers to the measurement taken when a child is standing upright. The child's shoes should be removed when measuring height. The head should be in midline and the child should be facing straight forward. There should be no flexion of the knees, slumping of the shoulders, or raising of the heels during the measurement. The most accurate measurements are taken with a wall-mounted stadiometer.

The nurse should use a balanced scale to measure a child's weight. Children should be weighed nude when using the birth to 36-month growth chart. If a child is wearing something heavy, such as a cast or an IV board, that should be documented with the child's weight. When placing the child on an infant scale, the nurse must remember safety issues.

Head circumference is another key growth measurement in children. In general, head circumference is measured from birth to 36 months of age. The measurement should be taken at the greatest circumference, which is slightly above the eyebrows and ear pinna and around the occipital prominence at the back of the skull. A paper tape measure should be used to give the most accurate data.

Chest circumference is measured primarily for comparison with head circumference. Chest circumference is measured at the nipple line midway between inspiration and expiration.

Measuring skinfold thickness is one way to assess body fat. Calipers are used to measure the skinfold thickness in one or more of the following sites: triceps, subscapula, abdomen, upper thigh, and suprailiac. An average of at least two measurements from each site is used.

The measurement of arm circumference is an indirect assessment used to evaluate nutrition. The arm circumference is measured with a paper tape measure, which is placed vertically along the posterior upper arm until the same measurement appears at the acromial process and olecranon process.

NORMAL GROWTH PARAMETERS RELATED TO WEIGHT, HEIGHT, AND HEAD CIRCUMFERENCE

Age	Weight	Height	Head Circumference
1–6 mo	Gains 5–8 oz per wk	Grows 1 inch per mo	
7–12 mo	Gains 4–5 oz per wk	Grows ½ inch per mo	
12–18 mo	Gains 2–6 lb in next 6 mo Average weight is 20–24 lb Birth weight is tripled by 12 mo	Grows to 33 inches by 18 mo	Head circumference equals chest circumference at 12 mo
18 mo–3 yr	Average weight is 28–30 lb Birth weight is quadrupled by 2 yr	Grows to 33–37 inches Approximately 50% of adult height by 2 yr	
3–6 yr	Average weight is 44 lb	Grows to 44 inches Birth length doubles by 4 yr Height and weight are even at 5 yr	
7–11 yr	Gains 5–7 lb per year	Growth appears in spurts Increases 3 inches per year to 52 inches at 7–10 yr	

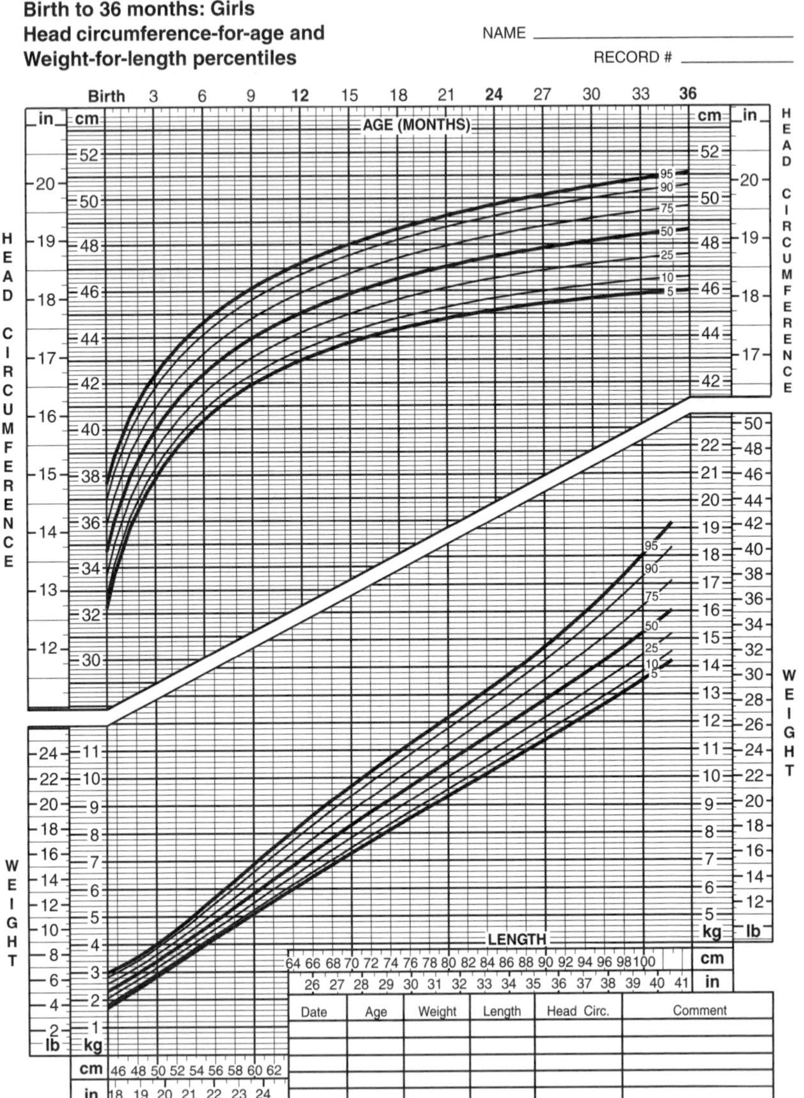

SOURCE: Developed by the National Center for Health Statistics in collaboration with the National Center for Chronic Disease Prevention and Health Promotion (2000). **http://www.cdc.gov/growthcharts**

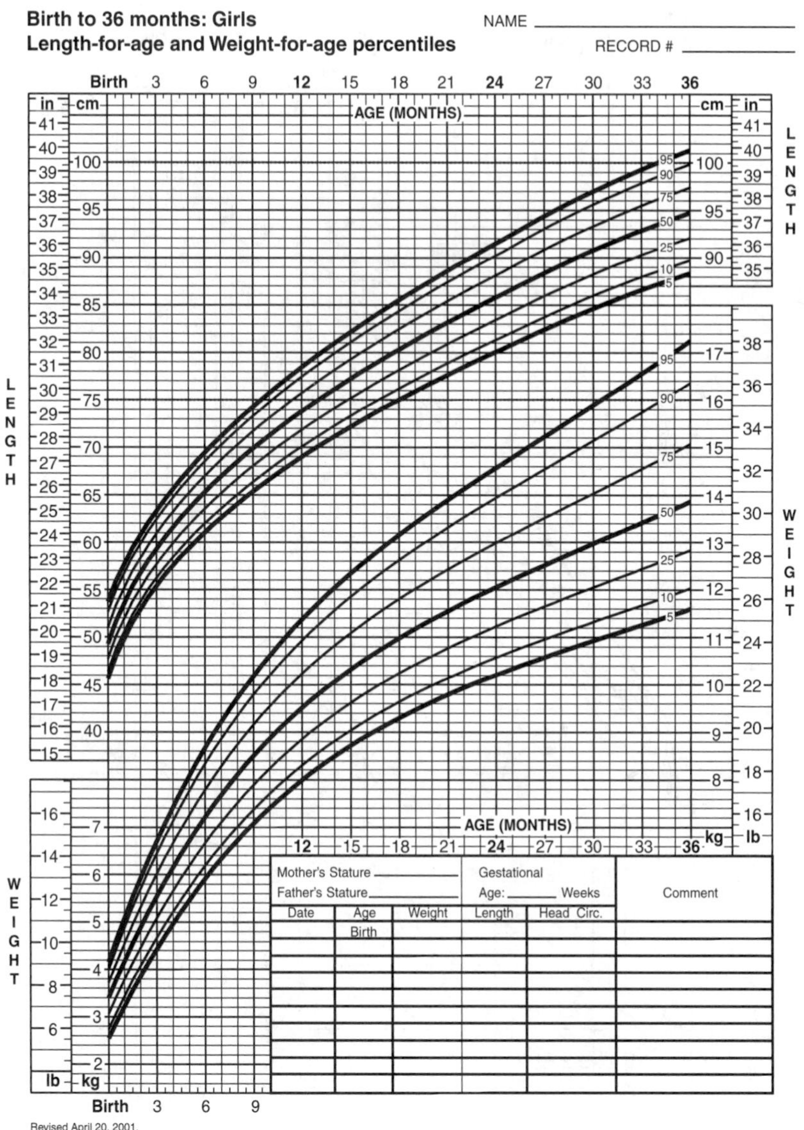

Revised April 20, 2001.
SOURCE: Developed by the National Center for Health Statistics in collaboration with the National Center for Chronic Disease Prevention and Health Promotion (2000).
http://www.cdc.gov/growthcharts

2 to 20 years: Girls
Stature-for-age and Weight-for-age percentiles

NAME ______________________

RECORD # ______________

Mother's Stature ____________ Father's Stature ____________

Date	Age	Weight	Stature	BMI*

***To Calculate BMI**: Weight (kg) ÷ Stature (cm) ÷ Stature (cm) x 10,000
or Weight (lb) ÷ Stature (in) ÷ Stature (in) x 703

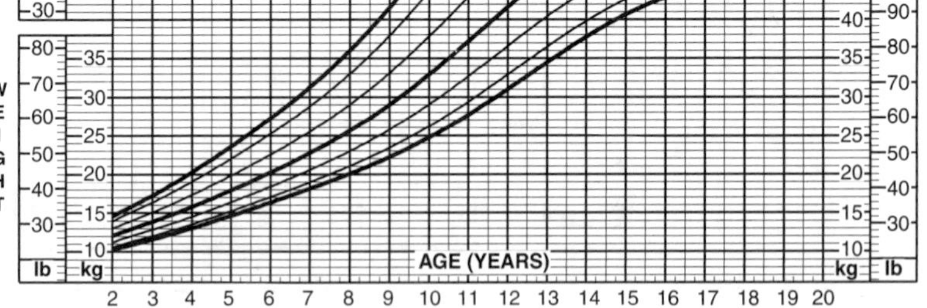

Revised and corrected November 21, 2000.
SOURCE: Developed by the National Center for Health Statistics in collaboration with
the National Center for Chronic Disease Prevention and Health Promotion (2000).
http://www.cdc.gov/growthcharts

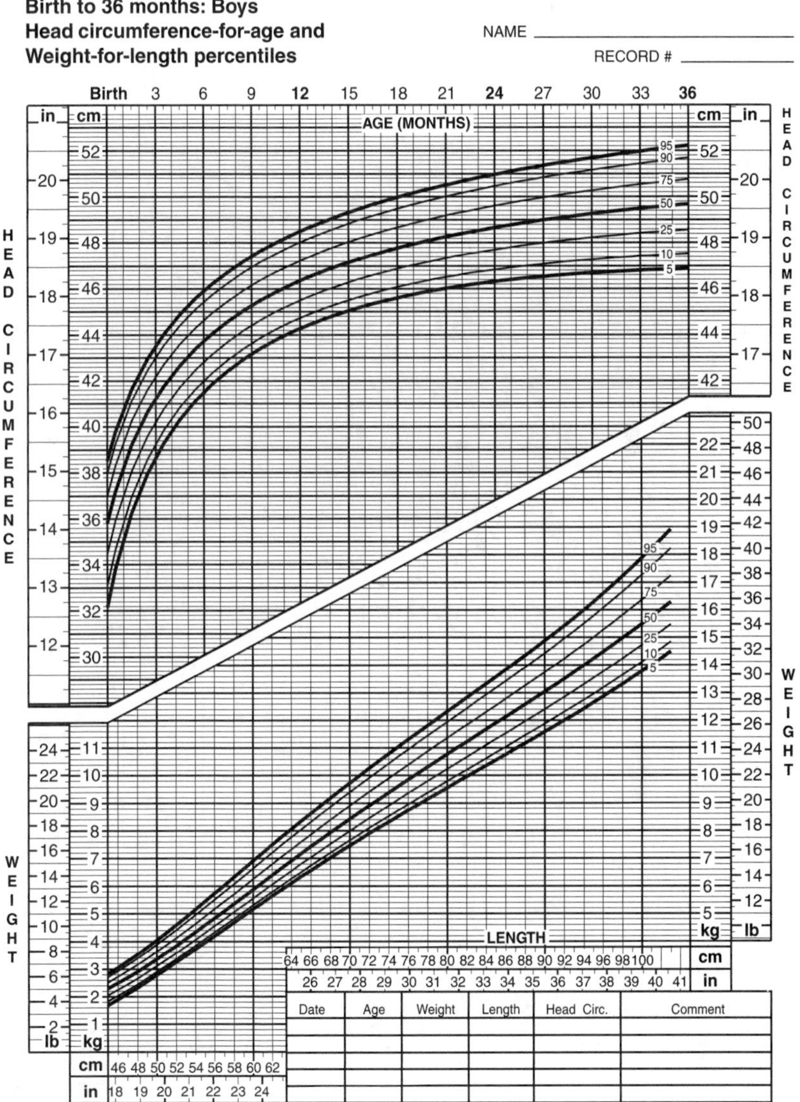

SOURCE: Developed by the National Center for Health Statistics in collaboration with the National Center for Chronic Disease Prevention and Health Promotion (2000). **http://www.cdc.gov/growthcharts**

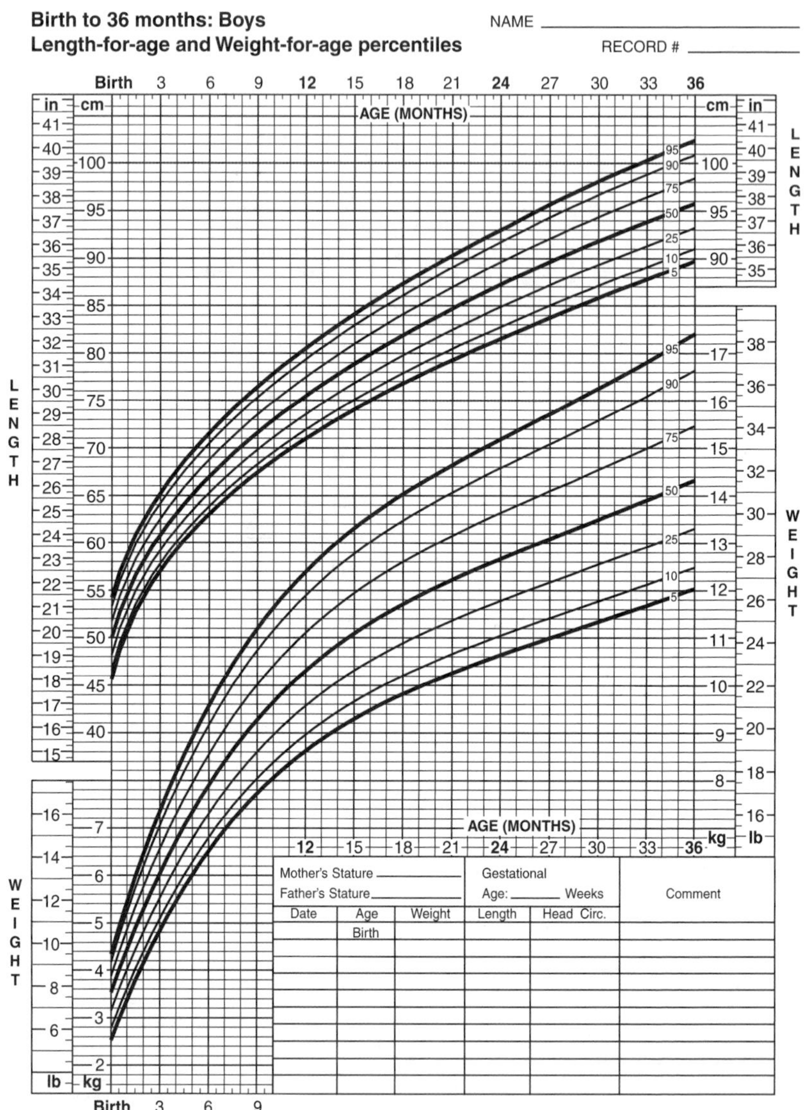

Revised April 20, 2001.
SOURCE: Developed by the National Center for Health Statistics in collaboration with the National Center for Chronic Disease Prevention and Health Promotion (2000).
http://www.cdc.gov/growthcharts

2 to 20 years: Boys
Stature-for-age and Weight-for-age percentiles

NAME ____________________

RECORD # __________

Mother's Stature ______________ Father's Stature ______________

Date	Age	Weight	Stature	BMI*

***To Calculate BMI**: Weight (kg) ÷ Stature (cm) ÷ Stature (cm) x 10,000
or Weight (lb) ÷ Stature (in) ÷ Stature (in) x 703

AGE (YEARS)

STATURE

WEIGHT

Revised and corrected November 21, 2000.

SOURCE: Developed by the National Center for Health Statistics in collaboration with the National Center for Chronic Disease Prevention and Health Promotion (2000).
http://www.cdc.gov/growthcharts

NUTRITIONAL ASSESSMENT

Nutritional status affects the general health of a child and has a direct influence on a child's growth, development, cognition, and learning. A nutritional assessment is an essential component of a complete health history. A complete nutritional assessment incorporates information about dietary intake, clinical assessment of nutritional status, and biochemical status.

A thorough dietary history should be obtained by the nurse. The following types of questions should be included in your assessment:

- Usual mealtimes
- Which family member is responsible for meal preparation and shopping
- How much money is allotted for groceries each week
- How most foods are prepared (e.g., baked, fried, broiled, microwaved)
- How often the family eats out (frequency of fast food restaurants)
- Favorite foods, snacks
- Cultural practices/ethnic foods
- Food/beverage dislikes
- Description of child's usual appetite
- Feeding habits
- Breastfeeding
- Past medical history including any emotional difficulties
- Medication history
- Supplemental vitamins, herbs, iron, fluoride
- Food allergies
- Special diets
- Recent weight gain/loss
- Types of routine exercise

Additional information to obtain for young infants includes the following:

- Birth history (e.g., birth weight, history of prematurity, small for gestational age)
- Past medical history, especially in terms of gastrointestinal disturbances
- Feeding difficulties such as excessive fussiness, colic, regurgitation, difficulty swallowing/sucking

Dietary Intake

A thorough diet history should be obtained by the nurse. Food intake can be recorded by using a food diary and/or a food frequency record.

Record the following types of information in a food diary:

- Times of meals and snacks
- Description of food items including the actual food, amount, and method of preparation

- With whom the child ate
- Related factors such as associated activity, place, persons, feelings, hunger

Record the following types of information in a food frequency record:

- Food group (breads/cereals/pasta, milk/cheese/yogurt, vegetables, fruits/juice, protein foods, fats/oils/sweets)
- Numbers of servings per day or week in each of the food groups
- Serving size

Clinical Assessment

Another component of the nutritional assessment is the clinical examination of the child. This provides information regarding signs of adequate nutrition or deficiencies. Assessment of the skin, hair, mouth, teeth, eyes, neck, chest, abdomen, cardiovascular system, neurological system, and musculoskeletal system can be useful in determining possible nutritional deficits or excesses (see table on page 30 for physical signs of nutritional deficits). Anthropomorphic measurements of height, weight, head circumference, skinfold thickness, and arm circumference are also essential components of the physical examination.

Biochemical Analysis

Biochemical analysis is the last integral component of the nutritional assessment. Blood chemistry levels of hematocrit and hemoglobin (indication of anemias), albumin (protein malnutrition), blood urea nitrogen (negative nitrogen balance), creatinine (high protein intake), lead (water consumption containing lead), glucose (dehydration, acidosis), and cholesterol (dietary-fat intake) should be analyzed. Normal values for these tests are located in Chapter 3.

CALCULATING DAILY CALORIC REQUIREMENTS

Body Weight (kg)	Caloric Expenditure/Day
Up to 10	100 kcal/kg
11–20	1,000 kcal + 50 kcal/kg for each kg above 10 kg
More than 20	1,500 kcal + 20 kcal/kg for each kg above 20 kg

These formulas are not appropriate for neonates less than 2 weeks old or for children with conditions associated with abnormal losses. In addition, children with disease, prior surgery, fever, or pain may require additional calories above the maintenance value. Children who are comatose or immobile may require fewer calories.

PHYSICAL SIGNS ASSOCIATED WITH NUTRITIONAL DEFICITS

Body Part	Normal Appearance	Physical Signs	Nutritional Deficit/ Excess
Skin	Uniform color, smooth, firm	Depigmentation, scaling, dry appearance, edema, pallor	Vitamin A, protein, riboflavin, vitamin B_{12}, excess sodium
Hair	Shiny, strong, not easily plucked	Dull, dry, thin, alopecia depigmentation	Protein, calories, vitamin C
Mouth	Lips smooth, pink, not chapped; tongue rough texture, no lesions; teeth white, no cavities; gums firm, pink; mucous membranes moist, pink, smooth	Lips reddened, swollen, cracked; tongue—glossitis; teeth brown, pitted, with caries; gums spongy, bleeding, swollen; mucous membranes with ulcers	Riboflavin, vitamin C, niacin, fluoride; excess carbohydrates, excess vitamin A
Eyes	Clear, bright, moist membranes	Pale conjunctiva, night blindness, corneal drying	Vitamin A, riboflavin
Neck	Thyroid not visible	Thyroid enlarged, grossly visible	Iodine
Chest	Chest is almost circular; lateral diameter increases in proportion to anteroposterior diameter in children	Depressed rib cage, protrusion of sternum	Vitamin D
Abdomen	Abdomen is slightly protruded; older children have flat abdomen	Abdominal distension, poor musculature	Protein, calories
Cardiovascular system	Heart rate and blood pressure within normal limits	Tachycardia, palpitations, arrhythmias, increased blood pressure	Potassium, magnesium; excess sodium
Neurological system	Alert, emotionally stable, intact reflexes	Irritable, listless, lethargic, diminished or absent deep tendon reflexes	Thiamin, niacin, vitamin C, vitamin E
Musculoskeletal system	Firm muscles, bilaterally equal strength, normal spinal curves, symmetric and straight extremities, full range of motion	Weak, wasting appearance, kyphosis/lordosis/scoliosis, bowing of extremities	Protein, calories, vitamin D, calcium, vitamin A

DEVELOPMENTAL ASSESSMENT

Children are at high risk for developmental delay and regression resulting from the stress of hospitalization. To most appropriately interact with children and to encourage their development, the nurse needs to be knowledgeable about normal growth and developmental milestones.

General Information

Patterns of development are sequential and predictable. Children must achieve one level before they can proceed to the next. Caregivers play an extremely important role in developmental assessment. Timing of speech and language development are most helpful in the determination of normalcy. Vision, hearing, and physical impairment, as well as illness and hospitalization, adversely affect the results of standardized developmental testing.

Developmental Characteristics

Infant (Birth to 1 year)–Erikson's Trust versus Mistrust

Personal/Social. Consistency of care is essential to the development of trust. Signaled needs must be met promptly and consistently.

Cognitive. The infant learns to separate self from other objects. The concept of object permanence, which develops at approximately 9 to 10 months, is necessary for the development of self-image.

Motor. The infant progresses from rolling over to reaching out to sitting to beginning to creep and crawl.

Toddler (1 to 3 years)–Erikson's Autonomy versus Shame and Doubt

Personal/Social. This is a period of holding on and letting go. Children begin to tolerate some separation from the parent. They engage in parallel play. Temper tantrums are an expression of frustration of not being able to verbalize wants. Children need rituals and a safe environment to develop autonomy. They use negativism in quest for autonomy.

Language/Cognitive. The major achievement is language development. Appearance of an object denotes function. Children imitate household activities, and are very egocentric.

Motor. A major skill is the development of locomotion (e.g., walking, running, climbing). A major task is toilet training. Children develop pincher grasp.

Preschooler (3 to 6 Years)–Erikson's Initiative versus Guilt

Personal/Social. Children need a security object. They are learning sex differences. They are energetic learners and feel guilt for not behaving or acting appropriately; they also may feel guilt from having thoughts that differ from the perceived norm. Beginnings of morality and the development of a conscience become evident. Children have a fear of mutilation and injury. They have poorly defined body boundaries and need a bandage to cover injuries to maintain body integrity.

Language/Cognitive. Preschoolers talk incessantly and in complete sentences. They have global organization of thought. Changing any part of something changes the whole thing. They give life-like qualities to inanimate objects. Preschoolers cannot perceive opposite behavior so caregivers need to phrase directions positively. They are shifting from total egocentricity to beginning to be able to consider other viewpoints. They have magical thinking and accept meaning literally.

Motor. Walking, running, climbing, and jumping are well established. Most children can use scissors by age 4 years and tie shoes by 5 years.

School-Aged Child (6 to 12 years)—Erikson's Industry versus Inferiority

Personal/Social. The goal is to achieve a sense of personal and interpersonal competence by acquiring technologies and social skills. Failure to accomplish this leads to a sense of inferiority. Further development of conscience occurs. Peer groups are influential and necessary but caregivers are still the primary influence.

Language/Cognitive. Children use thought processes to explore events. They can see things from other points of view, and can reason. They are present-oriented and learn best with concrete examples.

Adolescent (12 to 18 years)—Erikson's Identity versus Role Confusion

Personal/Social. Adolescents are trying to develop a sense of identity. Early adolescents need peer approval; peer pressure may lead to risk taking behaviors. Late adolescents need autonomy from their family and develop a sense of personal identity. They need a group identity to develop a personal identity. They are on an emotional roller coaster. Body image established during adolescence is retained throughout life.

Cognitive. Adolescents can think beyond the present and are concerned with the possible. Adolescents use logic and scientific reasoning, and are capable of abstract thinking. They want a clear picture of life and its purposes. They often believe they are invincible.

Developmental Assessment Tools

Optimum developmental screening should be done with healthy, nonhospitalized children. Children who are hospitalized may have multiple variables interfering with normal testing. There are many tools available. The most commonly used tool is the Denver II Developmental Screening Test. Although during hospitalization is not the optimum time to test children, this tool can be used as a quick reference for the sequencing of normal milestones and to help identify areas that would be appropriate for stimulation.

Denver II Developmental Screening Test

The Denver II is used to assess well children from birth to 6 years of age. It is designed to "compare a given child's performance on a variety of tasks to the performance of other children the same age" (Frankenburg & Dodds, 1990). It is not a predictor of future development and does not test intelligence quotient. To perform the Denver II, the nurse must be trained, must follow strict guidelines that are specific to testing and interpretation, and must use the kit with the materials provided. The Denver II assesses development in four general areas. The Denver II test follows, concluding with a summary of milestones assessed on the Denver II to assist the nurse in assessing and encouraging normal development in hospitalized children.

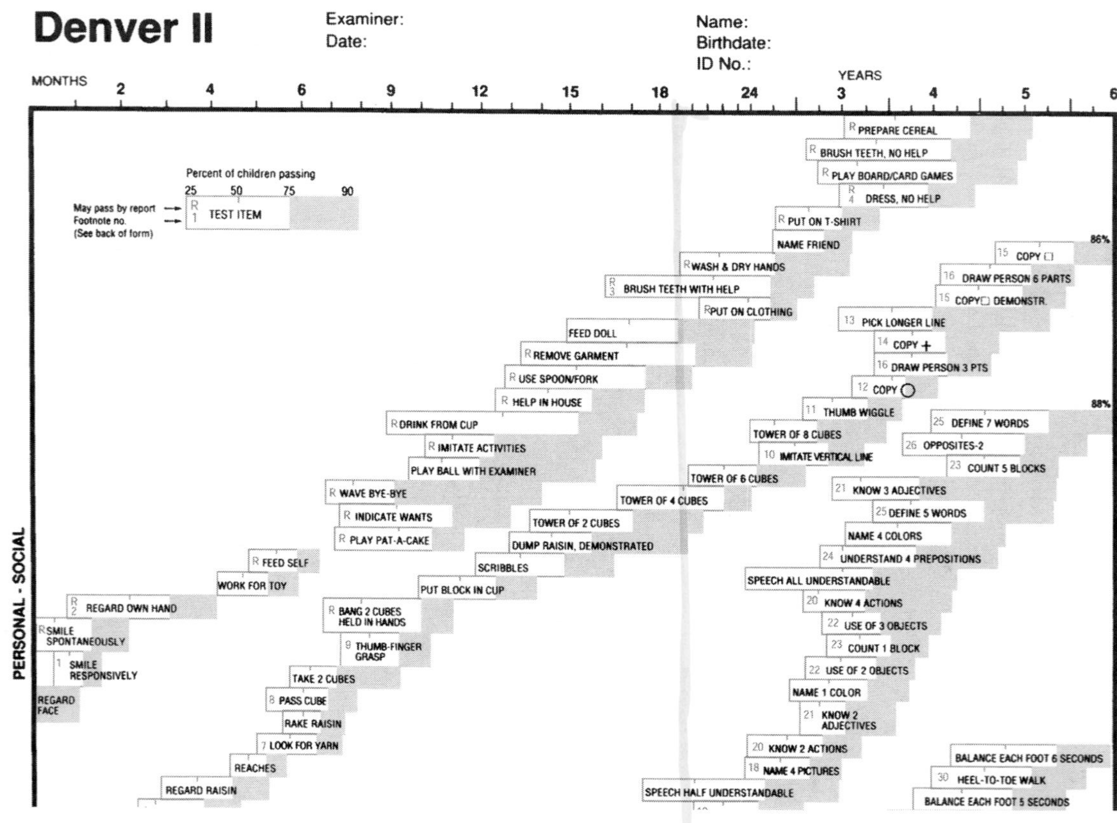
Denver II
Examiner:
Date:
Name:
Birthdate:
ID No.:
MONTHS 2 4 6 9 12 15 18 24
YEARS 3 4 5 6
Percent of children passing
25 50 75 90
May pass by report
Footnote no.
(See back of form)
R 1 TEST ITEM
R PREPARE CEREAL
R BRUSH TEETH, NO HELP
R PLAY BOARD/CARD GAMES
R 4 DRESS, NO HELP
R PUT ON T-SHIRT
NAME FRIEND
R WASH & DRY HANDS
R 3 BRUSH TEETH WITH HELP
R PUT ON CLOTHING
FEED DOLL
R REMOVE GARMENT
R USE SPOON/FORK
R HELP IN HOUSE
R DRINK FROM CUP
R IMITATE ACTIVITIES
PLAY BALL WITH EXAMINER
R WAVE BYE-BYE
R INDICATE WANTS
R PLAY PAT-A-CAKE
R FEED SELF
WORK FOR TOY
R 2 REGARD OWN HAND
R SMILE SPONTANEOUSLY
1 SMILE RESPONSIVELY
REGARD FACE
PERSONAL - SOCIAL
86%
15 COPY □
16 DRAW PERSON 6 PARTS
15 COPY□ DEMONSTR.
13 PICK LONGER LINE
14 COPY +
16 DRAW PERSON 3 PTS
12 COPY ○
11 THUMB WIGGLE
TOWER OF 8 CUBES
10 IMITATE VERTICAL LINE
TOWER OF 6 CUBES
TOWER OF 4 CUBES
TOWER OF 2 CUBES
DUMP RAISIN, DEMONSTRATED
SCRIBBLES
PUT BLOCK IN CUP
R BANG 2 CUBES HELD IN HANDS
9 THUMB-FINGER GRASP
TAKE 2 CUBES
8 PASS CUBE
RAKE RAISIN
7 LOOK FOR YARN
REACHES
REGARD RAISIN
88%
25 DEFINE 7 WORDS
26 OPPOSITES-2
23 COUNT 5 BLOCKS
21 KNOW 3 ADJECTIVES
25 DEFINE 5 WORDS
NAME 4 COLORS
24 UNDERSTAND 4 PREPOSITIONS
SPEECH ALL UNDERSTANDABLE
20 KNOW 4 ACTIONS
22 USE OF 3 OBJECTS
23 COUNT 1 BLOCK
22 USE OF 2 OBJECTS
NAME 1 COLOR
21 KNOW 2 ADJECTIVES
20 KNOW 2 ACTIONS
18 NAME 4 PICTURES
SPEECH HALF UNDERSTANDABLE
BALANCE EACH FOOT 6 SECONDS
30 HEEL-TO-TOE WALK
BALANCE EACH FOOT 5 SECONDS

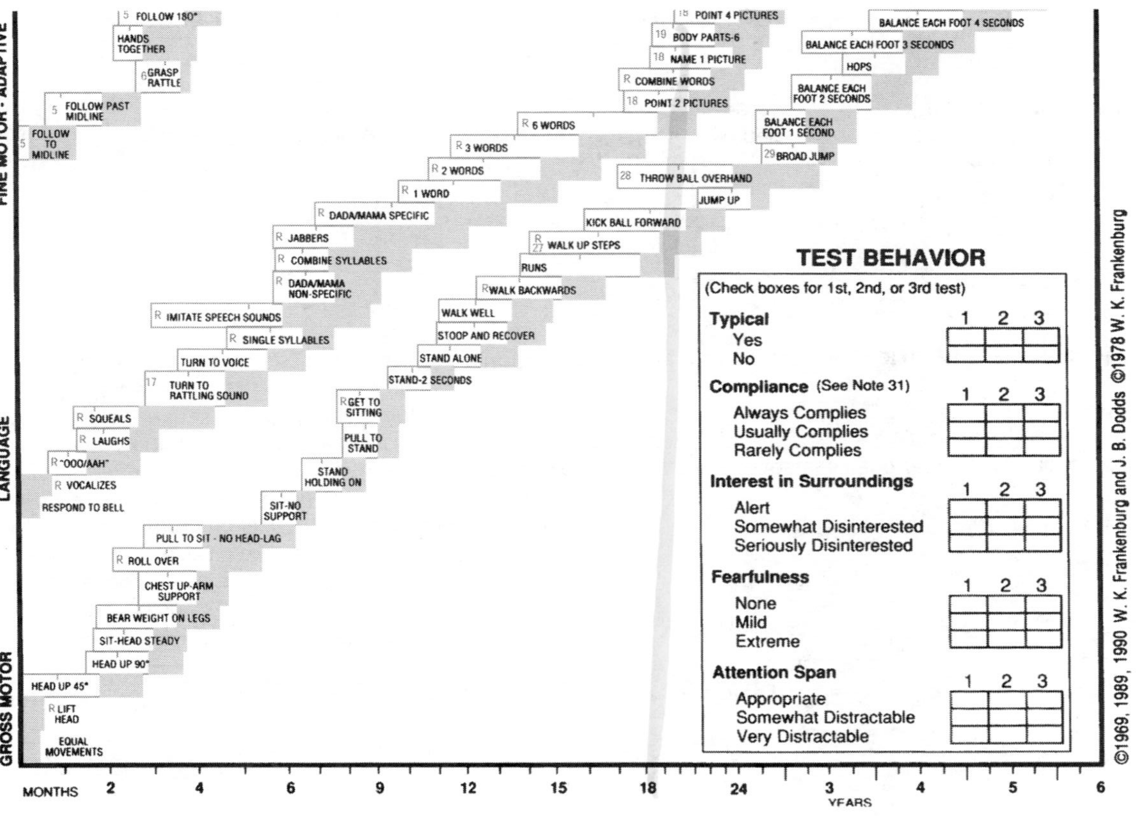

FINE MOTOR - ADAPTIVE
LANGUAGE
GROSS MOTOR
FOLLOW 180°
HANDS TOGETHER
GRASP RATTLE
FOLLOW PAST MIDLINE
FOLLOW TO MIDLINE
POINT 4 PICTURES
BODY PARTS-6
NAME 1 PICTURE
COMBINE WORDS
POINT 2 PICTURES
6 WORDS
3 WORDS
2 WORDS
1 WORD
DADA/MAMA SPECIFIC
JABBERS
COMBINE SYLLABLES
DADA/MAMA NON-SPECIFIC
IMITATE SPEECH SOUNDS
SINGLE SYLLABLES
TURN TO VOICE
TURN TO RATTLING SOUND
SQUEALS
LAUGHS
"OOO/AAH"
VOCALIZES
RESPOND TO BELL
BALANCE EACH FOOT 4 SECONDS
BALANCE EACH FOOT 3 SECONDS
HOPS
BALANCE EACH FOOT 2 SECONDS
BALANCE EACH FOOT 1 SECOND
BROAD JUMP
THROW BALL OVERHAND
JUMP UP
KICK BALL FORWARD
WALK UP STEPS
RUNS
WALK BACKWARDS
WALK WELL
STOOP AND RECOVER
STAND ALONE
STAND-2 SECONDS
GET TO SITTING
PULL TO STAND
STAND HOLDING ON
SIT-NO SUPPORT
PULL TO SIT - NO HEAD-LAG
ROLL OVER
CHEST UP-ARM SUPPORT
BEAR WEIGHT ON LEGS
SIT-HEAD STEADY
HEAD UP 90°
HEAD UP 45°
LIFT HEAD
EQUAL MOVEMENTS
TEST BEHAVIOR
(Check boxes for 1st, 2nd, or 3rd test)
Typical
Yes
No
Compliance (See Note 31)
Always Complies
Usually Complies
Rarely Complies
Interest in Surroundings
Alert
Somewhat Disinterested
Seriously Disinterested
Fearfulness
None
Mild
Extreme
Attention Span
Appropriate
Somewhat Distractable
Very Distractable
1 2 3
MONTHS 2 4 6 9 12 15 18 24 3 4 5 6
YEARS
©1969, 1989, 1990 W. K. Frankenburg and J. B. Dodds ©1978 W. K. Frankenburg

DIRECTIONS FOR ADMINISTRATION

1. Try to get child to smile by smiling, talking or waving. Do not touch him/her.
2. Child must stare at hand several seconds.
3. Parent may help guide toothbrush and put toothpaste on brush.
4. Child does not have to be able to tie shoes or button/zip in the back.
5. Move yarn slowly in an arc from one side to the other, about 8" above child's face.
6. Pass if child grasps rattle when it is touched to the backs or tips of fingers.
7. Pass if child tries to see where yarn went. Yarn should be dropped quickly from sight from tester's hand without arm movement.
8. Child must transfer cube from hand to hand without help of body, mouth, or table.
9. Pass if child picks up raisin with any part of thumb and finger.
10. Line can vary only 30 degrees or less from tester's line.
11. Make a fist with thumb pointing upward and wiggle only the thumb. Pass if child imitates and does not move any fingers other than the thumb.

12. Pass any enclosed form. Fail continuous round motions.
13. Which line is longer? (Not bigger.) Turn paper upside down and repeat. (pass 3 of 3 or 5 of 6)
14. Pass any lines crossing near midpoint.
15. Have child copy first. If failed, demonstrate.

When giving items 12, 14, and 15, do not name the forms. Do not demonstrate 12 and 14.

16. When scoring, each pair (2 arms, 2 legs, etc.) counts as one part.
17. Place one cube in cup and shake gently near child's ear, but out of sight. Repeat for other ear.
18. Point to picture and have child name it. (No credit is given for sounds only.)
    If less than 4 pictures are named correctly, have child point to picture as each is named by tester.

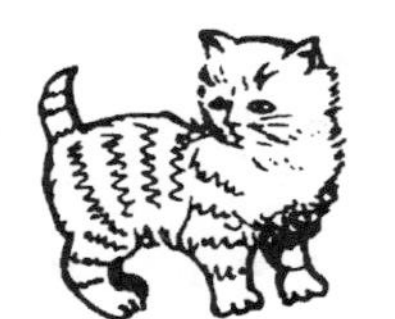 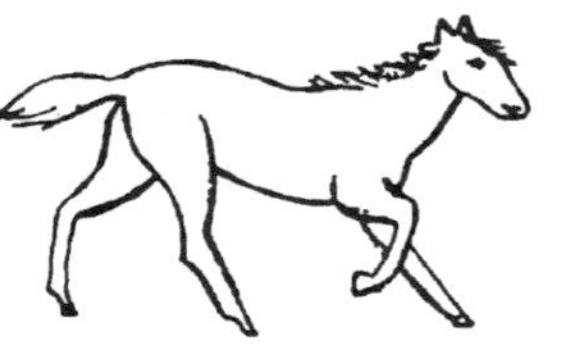 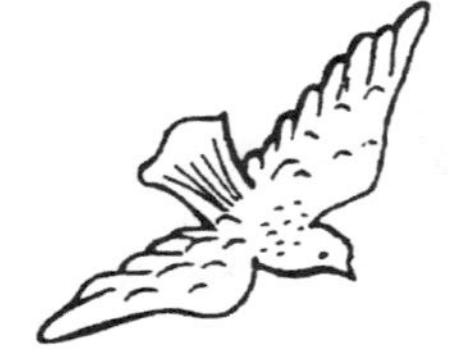 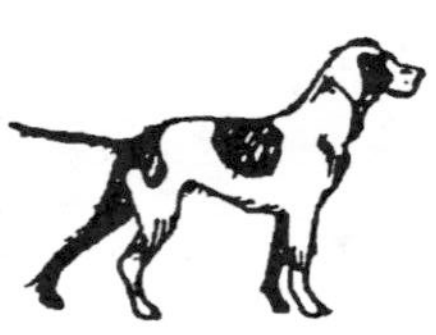 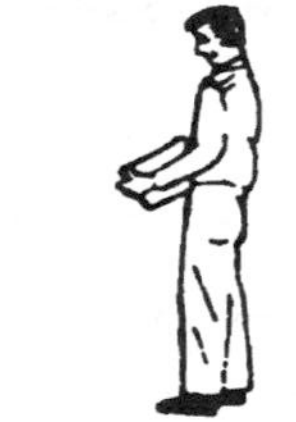

19. Using doll, tell child: Show me the nose, eyes, ears, mouth, hands, feet, tummy, hair. Pass 6 of 8.
20. Using pictures, ask child: Which one flies?... says meow?... talks?... barks?... gallops? Pass 2 of 5, 4 of 5.
21. Ask child: What do you do when you are cold?... tired?... hungry? Pass 2 of 3, 3 of 3.
22. Ask child: What do you do with a cup? What is a chair used for? What is a pencil used for?
    Action words must be included in answers.
23. Pass if child correctly places <u>and</u> says how many blocks are on paper. (1, 5).
24. Tell child: Put block **on** table; **under** table; **in front of** me, **behind** me. Pass 4 of 4.
    (Do not help child by pointing, moving head or eyes.)
25. Ask child: What is a ball?... lake?... desk?... house?... banana?... curtain?... fence?... ceiling? Pass if defined in terms of use, shape, what it is made of, or general category (such as banana is fruit, not just yellow). Pass 5 of 8, 7 of 8.
26. Ask child: If a horse is big, a mouse is __? If fire is hot, ice is __? If the sun shines during the day, the moon shines during the __? Pass 2 of 3.
27. Child may use wall or rail only, not person. May not crawl.
28. Child must throw ball overhand 3 feet to within arm's reach of tester.
29. Child must perform standing broad jump over width of test sheet (8 1/2 inches).
30. Tell child to walk forward, → heel within 1 inch of toe. Tester may demonstrate.
    Child must walk 4 consecutive steps.
31. In the second year, half of normal children are non-compliant.

OBSERVATIONS:

DEVELOPMENTAL GUIDELINES: DENVER II

Age	Personal/Social	Fine Motor/Adaptive	Language	Gross Motor
Birth	Regards face	—	Vocalizes; responds to bell	Lifts head, equal movements
2 mo	Spontaneous and responsive smile	Follows person or object to midline	Makes ooh/ah sounds	Lifts head 30–45 degrees
4 mo	Looks at hand	Grasps rattle; holds hands together	Laughs; squeals	Lifts head up 90 degrees; sits with head steady; begins to bear weight
6 mo	Works for toy	Follows person or object 180 degrees; looks at small objects; reaches	Turns toward rattling sound	Chest up, arms supportive; rolls over; pulls to sit; no head lag
9 mo	Feeds self	Develops object permanence; passes block from hand to hand; holds block in each hand	Turns toward voice; uses single syllables; imitates sounds "Dada/Mama" nonspecific	Sits with no support; stands holding on to support
12 mo	Plays pat-a-cake; indicates wants; waves bye-bye	Develops thumb-finger grasp; bangs two objects together	Combines syllables; jabbers	Pulls to stand; gets to sitting; stands 2 sec
15 mo	Begins to play ball; imitates activities; drinks from cup	Puts objects in cup	"Dada/Mama" specific plus knows one to two words	Stands alone; stoops, recovers; walks well
18 mo	Can use spoon	Scribbles; dumps things; builds a tower of two blocks	Knows two to six words	Walks backward; runs
2 yr	Removes own clothes	Builds a tower of two to four blocks	Knows six or more words; combines words	Runs well; walks up steps; kicks ball
3 yr	Puts on own clothes; washes and dries hands; brushes teeth with help	Builds a tower of six blocks	Knows six body parts; speech half understandable	Throws ball overhand; jumps up
4 yr	Puts on T-shirt	Builds tower of eight blocks; imitates vertical line; wiggles thumb	Names one color; counts 1 block; speech all understandable	Can do broad jump; balances for 2 sec on each foot
5 yr	Gets dressed without help	Draws three-part person; copies a "+"	Names four colors; understands "on," "under," "in front of," "behind"	Hops; balances for 3–4 sec on each foot
6 yr	Prepares cereal; brushes teeth with no help	Draws six-part person; copies a square; picks larger line	Knows cold, tired, hungry; counts five blocks; knows opposites	Walks heel-to-toe; balances for 6 sec on each foot

Revised Prescreening Developmental Questionnaire

The revised prescreening developmental questionnaire (R-PDQ) is a parent-answered prescreening questionnaire based on questions from the Denver II. It is used to assess children from birth to 6 years of age; four different forms are available based on age. This questionnaire gives the caregiver's perspective of the child's developmental abilities.

(Both of the aforementioned tests, with forms and complete instructions, are available from Denver Developmental Materials, Inc., P.O. Box 371075, Denver, CO 80237-5075; phone 800-419-4729.)

PAIN ASSESSMENT

Factors That Affect Children's Response to Pain

Culture
Developmental level
Caregiver attitudes
Expectations
Education/teaching
Type of anesthetic/procedure
Previous experience with pain
Caregiver's presence or absence
Nurse's/doctor's attitudes and beliefs about pain
Fear

Possible Physical Signs and Symptoms of Pain

Facial expression of discomfort/grimacing/crying
Immobility/guarding area of body
Elevated pulse/respirations
Irritability/restlessness
Decreased appetite
Crying

Developmental Responses to Pain

Infants. Irritability, crying, withdrawal, pushing away, restless sleeping, poor feeding.

Toddlers. Very quiet, regressive behavior, uncooperative, crying, pointing to where it hurts (more accurate in pointing to where it hurts than saying where it hurts), say "ooww," fear responses. (May leave room to go to safe area of the playroom even though he or she hurts because the fear of what will happen in the room overshadows the pain.)

Preschoolers. Become quiet, may feel pain is punishment for bad behavior or thoughts. Good at procrastination before painful procedures (persistent "Wait a minute" or "I have to go to the bathroom"). May be able to tell where it hurts and use tools to describe the severity.

School-Aged Children. May deny pain to be brave or to avoid further hurt. May withdraw, watch or stare at the television.

Adolescents. Fear loss of control. Are affected by mood changes and expectations of behavior. May refuse or over request medication. Show increased muscle tension.

Assessment Guidelines

Assess frequently and uniformly using age appropriate tools and nursing observations. Tools help to more accurately assess and record pain assessment and need to be used and recorded at least once a shift and 30 minutes to an hour after pain-relief method is applied or pain medication is given. This provides a record to determine whether pain is increasing or decreasing and whether relief methods are effective.

Consult hospital/institutional policy regarding tools used in your facility and read original information and guidelines for their use.

Pain Assessment Tools

Wong-Baker FACES Pain Scale.

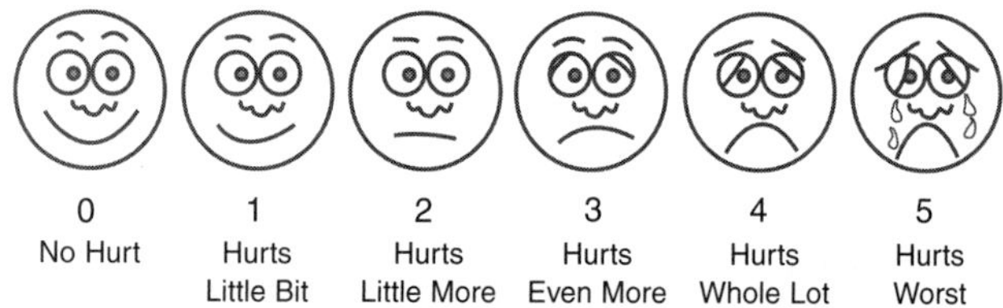

0	1	2	3	4	5
No Hurt	Hurts Little Bit	Hurts Little More	Hurts Even More	Hurts Whole Lot	Hurts Worst

Explain to the person that each face is for a person who feels happy because he has no pain (hurt) or sad because he has some or a lot of pain. Face) is very happy because he doesn't hurt at all. Face 1 hurts just a little bit. Face 2 hurts a little more. Face 3 hurts even more. Face 4 hurts a whole lot. Face 5 hurts as much as you can imagine, although you don't have to be crying to feel this bad. Ask the person to choose the face that best describes how he is feeling.

Rating scale is recommended for persons age 3 years and older.

From *Essentials of Pediatric Nursing* (p. 1301), by D. L. Wong, M. Hockenberry-Eaton, D, Wilson, M. L. Winkelstein, P. Schwartz, 2001, St. Louis: Mosby. Copyright 2001 by Mosby, Inc. Reprinted with permission.

This pain assessment tool can be used with children as young as 3 years.

Numeric scale. The numeric scale rates pain from 0 to 10, where 0 is no hurt, and 10 is worst hurt ever experienced. Child picks a number between 0 and 10 to describe the severity of hurt. The child must know numbers; this works best with children ages 5 years and older.

Poker Chip Tool. This tool uses five poker chips to measure pieces of hurt. Works best with children ages 4 years and older.

Color tool. This tool uses an outline of the body. The child chooses a color to indicate the degree of hurt and colors where it hurts.

ASSESSING LEVEL OF CONSCIOUSNESS IN CHILDREN

The Glasgow Coma Scale (GCS) is a standardized, objective assessment tool used to assess level of consciousness (LOC) in children. Nurses use their observational skills in three areas: eye opening, verbal response, and motor response. A value of 1 to 5 is assigned to each of the three areas. The sum of these numerical values is the objective measurement used to report LOC. A child with a score of 15 (highest) represents unaltered LOC. The lowest score of 3 represents deep coma or death. A score of 8 or less generally represents a comatose state. The pediatric version of the GCS recognizes the developmental variations among children of different ages in relation to expected verbal and motor responses.

MODIFIED PEDIATRIC GLASGOW COMA SCALE

		Score	
Eye opening	Spontaneously	4	
	To speech	3	
	To pain	2	
	None	1	
Best motor response (usually record best arm or age-appropriate response)	Obeys commands	6	
	Localizes pain	5	
	Flexion withdrawal	4	
	Flexion abnormal	3	
	Extension	2	
	None	1	
	Younger than 2 yr		**Older than 2 yr**
Best response to auditory and/or visual stimulus	Oriented	5	Smiles, listens, follows
	Confused	4	Cries, consolable
	Inappropriate words	3	Inappropriate persistent cry
	Incomprehensible words	2	Agitated, restless
	None	1	None
	Endotracheal tube	T	
	Coma Scale Total	_____	

ASSESSMENT AND CARE OF THE ORTHOPEDIC PATIENT

Cast Care

Remember that Plaster-of-Paris casts can take from 10 to 72 hours to dry completely.

Remember that fiberglass and other synthetic materials dry within 30 minutes.

Expose cast to air until dry.

Handle wet casts with palms of hands to prevent denting it with the fingers.

Check movement, sensation, pulses, and capillary refill of distal digits and compare bilaterally.

Elevate casted extremity to decrease swelling.

Keep small items that could be placed in the cast away from small children.

Use ice packs to help with itching and swelling.

Assess and medicate for pain as needed.

Traction Care

Assess alignment and pull.

Assess skin integrity under bandages for skin traction; change as needed when permitted.

Check pin sites in skeletal traction frequently for infection and bleeding. Clean and dress as ordered.

Assess neurovascular status as described in the physical examination section of this text.

Make sure ropes and pulleys are in original position and in good condition.

Keep bed in position ordered for desired pull.

Ensure ordered weight and keep weights hanging freely and out of traffic paths.

Provide pressure-reducing mattress.

Assess for skin breakdown in pressure areas.

Assess and medicate for pain as needed.

ASSESSMENT AND CARE OF THE POSTOPERATIVE PATIENT

Prepare the client's room for his or her return by turning bed down and ensuring that any pumps or suction equipment, emesis basin, or other needed equipment is ready.
Receive the client from recovery room.
Review orders and operation note.
Check vital signs immediately and as ordered, usually at least every 4 hours.
Assess skin color and turgor.
Assess level of consciousness.
Assess for pain routinely; document assessment and medicate as needed.
Check dressing and reinforce as needed; mark outline of discharge or bleeding on dressing.
Assess for bleeding elsewhere.
Check for bowel sounds.
Assess for bladder distention.
Keep accurate record of intake and output.
Encourage the client to turn, cough, and breathe deeply as condition permits.
Splint incision before encouraging coughing.
Report any excessive bleeding or abnormal vital signs.

ASSESSMENT OF SEXUAL MATURATION

The predictable development of secondary sexual characteristics during puberty is divided into five phases termed *Tanner stages*. Although the order of this development is predictable, the ages at which these changes occur varies.

Sexual Maturity in Females

Externally examine the female for secondary sexual characteristic development. Specifically, growth of breast tissue and public hair are assessed. The onset of breast development and pubic hair growth occurs between the ages of 8½ to 13 years old. The progression between stages 2 and 5 usually takes an average of 3 years. Menarche usually occurs during breast stage 3 or 4.

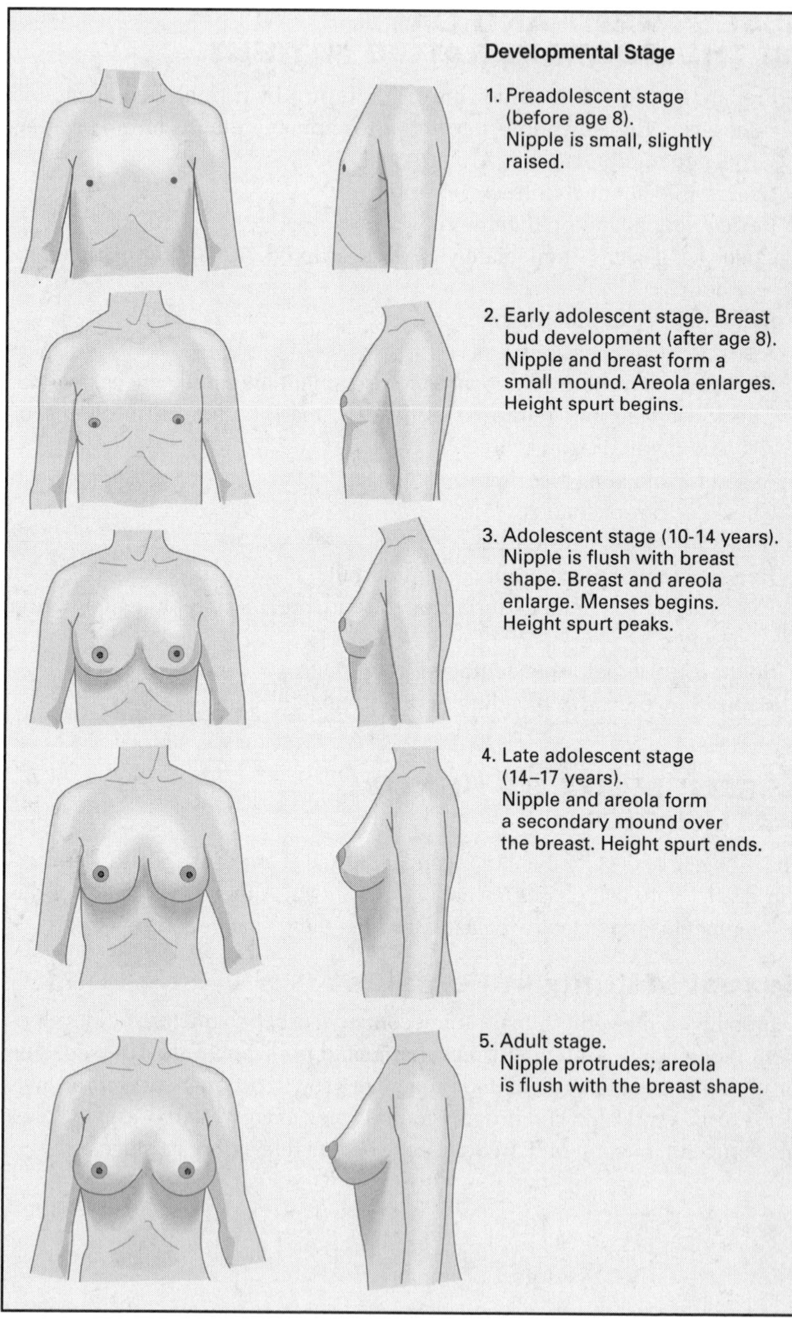
Developmental Stage
1. Preadolescent stage (before age 8). Nipple is small, slightly raised.
2. Early adolescent stage. Breast bud development (after age 8). Nipple and breast form a small mound. Areola enlarges. Height spurt begins.
3. Adolescent stage (10-14 years). Nipple is flush with breast shape. Breast and areola enlarge. Menses begins. Height spurt peaks.
4. Late adolescent stage (14–17 years). Nipple and areola form a secondary mound over the breast. Height spurt ends.
5. Adult stage. Nipple protrudes; areola is flush with the breast shape.

Stage 1

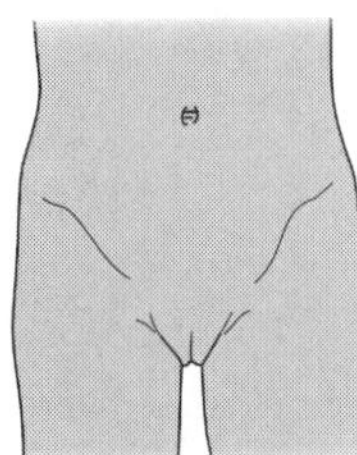

Preadolescent Stage
(before age 8)
No pubic hair, only body hair (vellus hair)

Stage 2

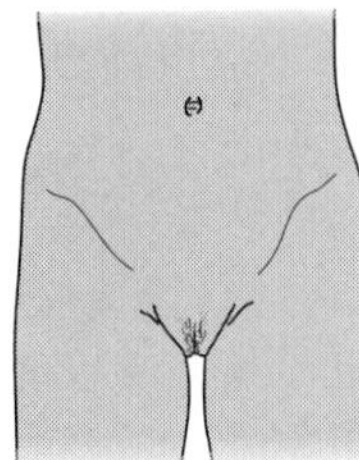

Early Adolescent Stage
(ages 8 to 12)
Sparse growth of long, slightly dark, fine pubic hair, slightly curly and located along the labia

Stage 3

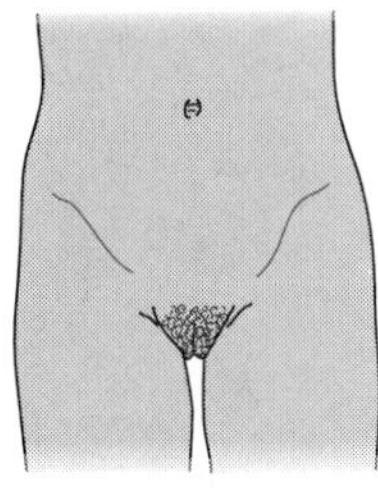

Adolescent Stage
(ages 12 to 13)
Pubic hair becomes darker, curlier, and spreads over the symphysis

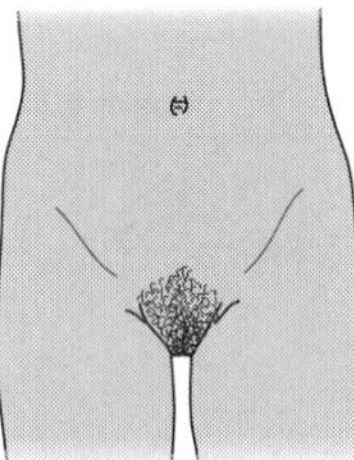

Late Adolescent Stage
(ages 13 to 15)
Texture and curl of pubic hair is similar to that of an adult but not spread to thighs

Stage 5

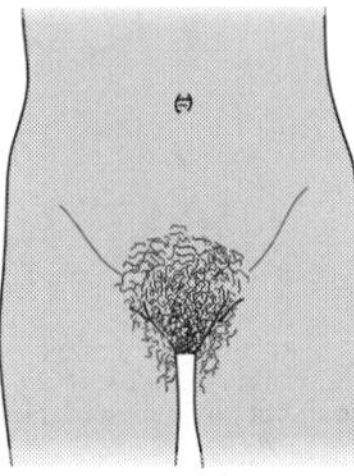

Adult Stage
Adult appearance in quality and quantity of pubic hair; growth is spread to inner aspect of thighs and abdomen

Sexual Maturity in Males

Externally examine the male for secondary sexual characteristic development. Specifically, growth of the testes and penis are assessed. The first changes in males are testicular enlargement with corresponding thinning, reddening, and loosening of the scrotum. This usually begins between 9½ to 13½ years of age. Maturation from preadolescent to adult usually occurs over a 3-year period.

1.		No pubic hair, only fine body hair (vellus hair)	Preadolescent; childhood size and proportion	Preadolescent; childhood size and proportion
2.	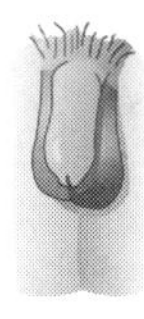	Sparse growth of long, slightly dark, straight hair	Slight or no growth	Growth in testes and scrotum; scrotum reddens and changes texture
3.	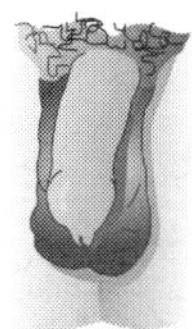	Becomes darker and coarser; slightly curled and spreads over symphysis	Growth, especially in length	Further growth
4.		Texture and curl of pubic hair is similar to that of an adult but not spread to thighs	Further growth in length; diameter increases; development of glans	Further growth; scrotum darkens
5.	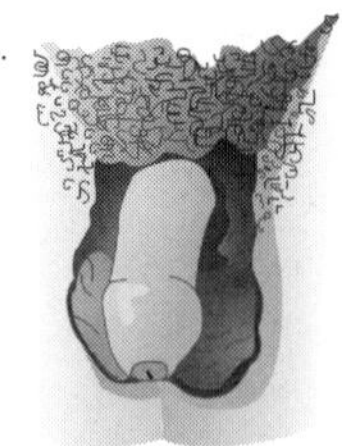	Adult appearance in quality and quantity of pubic hair; growth is spread to medial surface of thighs	Adult size and shape	Adult size and shape

ASSESSMENT FOR CHILD ABUSE

Failure to Thrive (nonorganic)

Lack of normal growth and development
Usually affects those 18 months and younger
Weight is below the 5th percentile
Is irritable, resists cuddling, and is unresponsive to nurturing
Appears thin, frail, undernourished
Has big, vacant eyes
May have gaze aversion
Has drawn, pinched, anxious or expressionless face; usually will not smile
Is obsessed with thumb or pacifier
Usually gains weight in hospital on same formula that he or she was on at home

Physical Abuse

Physical abuse is characterized by certain types of behaviors and injuries.

Behaviors Suspicious of Abuse

The following are characteristic behaviors typical of a child who is abused:

Withdrawn
Does not cry or respond to painful procedures
May accuse adult
May try to console the caregiver

Some characteristic behaviors of the caregiver of an abused child are as follows:

Delays seeking treatment
Is unable to comfort child
Decreases number of visits
Lacks follow-through
Blames child or child's sibling

In addition, there may be a variation in the child's history, the injury does not fit the history, and the accused caregiver is absent from visits.

Injuries Suspicious of Abuse

Bruises over soft tissue areas
Multiple planes of bruises
Multiple ages of bruises

Approximate dating of bruises (related to hemoglobin breakdown)

0–2 days	swollen and tender
0–5 days	red–blue
5–7 days	greenish yellow

7–10 days	yellow to brown
10–14 days	brown
2–4 weeks	clear

Fractures of different ages
Bilateral black eyes including upper lids
Slap, grab marks
Human bite marks with greater than 3 cm between canines (consistent with adult teeth)
Linear bruises from belt
Bruises shaped like the object used to inflict them
Tie marks on extremities
Gag marks
Cigarette burns
Dry contact burns that are second degree
Forced immersion burns (dunking or donut burns)—the buttocks and feet are usually spared because they were held against the cool bottom of the tub; there are no splash marks; and there is a clear line of demarcation between burned and unburned areas of skin
Stocking or glove burns with no splash marks—usually are clearly demarcated and go above the ankle or the wrist
Subdural hematomas with retinal hemorrhages from a shaking injury
Boggy scalp resulting from subgaleal hematomas caused by lifting the scalp off the skull
Traumatic alopecia/hair loss with tender scalp and broken hairs around patch of missing hair
Spiral fractures of the humerus or femur from a twisting injury
Fractured ribs in an infant
Bucket-handle fracture (chipped metaphysis) of femur or humerus, occurring because the child's ligaments are stronger than his or her bones

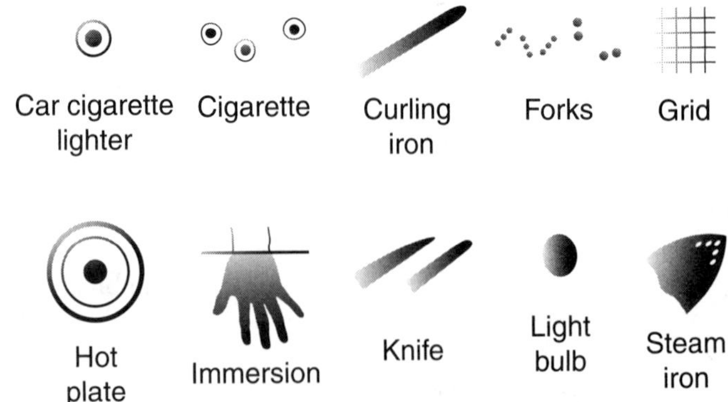

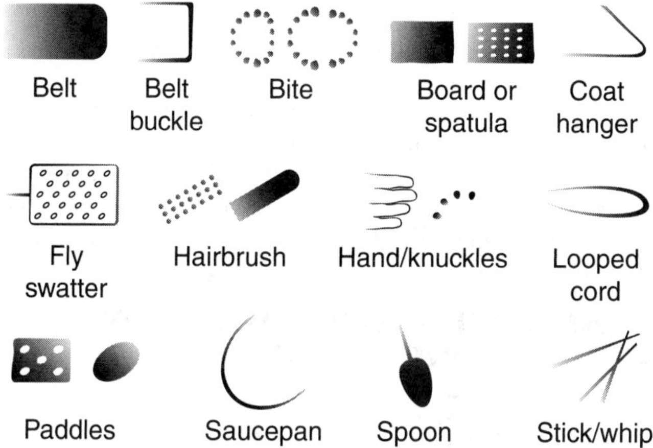

Signs of Sexual Abuse

Usually, few physical signs are present, but the following may be observed:

Abdominal and/or genital bruising
Lacerations of vagina or rectum
Sexually transmitted diseases in prepubertal child
Genital irritation or pain
Pregnancy

The following are behavioral signs typical of sexual abuse:

Advanced knowledge of explicit sexual behavior
Sexual acting out
Withdrawal
Fear of adult males or females
Depression
Encopresis (incontinence of stool)
Enuresis (incontinence of urine)
Runaway behaviors

The child's story often is the only evidence of the abuse. The nurse must believe the child. Abused children need support and, most importantly, need to know that the abuse is not in any way their fault. The guilt is tremendous and they need praise for having the courage to tell.

Munchausen Syndrome by Proxy

Child is usually 6 years old or younger
Child's signs and symptoms cannot be explained by known disease etiologies

Tests, X-ray films, and studies are negative
Child has repeated hospitalizations for the same problem
Perpetrator is usually the mother
Mother's history is unsupported by other caregivers
Child improves when mother is not present
Possible positive family history, especially siblings with same problems
Mother is overinvolved and has some type of experience in health care
Father is absent or uninvolved

SIGNS AND SYMPTOMS OF ILLICIT DRUG EXPOSURE OR USE

Neonatal Exposure

Symmetrical growth retardation, decreased weight and FOC
Poor response to auditory and visual stimuli, may be sleepy and/or easily overstimulated and may become irritable
Poor feeding versus hyperphagia (rapidly sucks down 3 to 4 oz at first feeding)
Vomiting/diarrhea
Sweating
Excessive crying/shrill cry/irritable
Jittery, has tremors
Hyperreflexia/increased muscle tone versus decreased muscle tone
Frantic hand sucking
Pallor
Poor sleeping
Frequent sneezing/yawning
Temperature instability
Seizure

Drug Use

Physical Signs and Symptoms (and Possible Drug Association)
Headache (inhalants)
Hyperreflexia (cocaine, hallucinogens)
Hyporeflexia (narcotics, heroin)
Slurred speech, ataxia (alcohol)
Bulky muscles (steroids)
Jaundice (alcohol)
Tachycardia, elevated blood pressure (alcohol, cocaine, hallucinogens)
Bradycardia, decreased blood pressure (heroin, narcotics)
Chest pain (cocaine)
Increased respirations (cocaine)

Decreased respirations (alcohol, heroin, narcotics)
Rhinorrhea (alcohol)
Erythematous nasal septum (cocaine, inhalants)
Epistaxis (cocaine)
Red, bloodshot eyes/conjunctivitis (alcohol, marijuana, inhalants)
Dilated pupils (cocaine)
Constricted pupils (heroin, narcotics)
Needle marks (heroin, narcotics)
Rapid precipitous delivery in primipara (cocaine)

Social Signs and Symptoms

Multiple accidents
Multiple sexually transmitted diseases
Aggressive behavior
Antisocial behavior

Psychologic Signs and Symptoms

Depression
Anxiety
Sleep changes
Hallucinations
Euphoria
Mood changes (excessive)
Memory loss/blackouts

CHAPTER 3

CLINICAL VALUES AND STANDARDS

CALCULATING DAILY MAINTENANCE FLUID REQUIREMENTS IN CHILDREN

Body weight (kg)	Amount of fluid per day
1–10 kg	100 mL/kg
11–20 kg	1,000 mL + 50 mL/kg for each kg more than 10 kg
>20 kg	1,500 mL + 20 mL/kg for each kg more than 20 kg

Urine output should average 0.5–1.0 mL/kg per hour when the child's fluid intake is adequate.

NORMAL LABORATORY VALUES AND INTERPRETATION

Acetaminophen

Therapeutic concentration	10–30 μg/mL
Toxic concentration	>200 μg/mL

Alanine Aminotransferase (ALT)/Serum Glutamic-pyruvic Transaminase (SGPT)

Infant	<54 U/L
Child/adult	1–30 U/L

- Major sources: liver, skeletal muscle, and myocardium
- Increased in severe hepatitis, infectious mononucleosis, congestive heart failure (CHF), and eclampsia
- Not as specific for liver function as aspartate aminotransferase (AST)

Aldolase

Newborn	<32 U/L
Child	<16 U/L
Adult	<8 U/L

- Major sources: skeletal muscle, myocardium, and liver
- Increased in muscular tissue damage and progressive muscular dystrophy
- Not increased in myasthenia gravis or multiple sclerosis

Alkaline Phosphatase

Infant	150–420 U/L
2–10 yr	100–320 U/L
11–18 yr (male)	100–390 U/L
11–18 yr (female)	100–320 U/L
Adult	30–120 U/L

- Major sources: bone, intestinal mucosa, liver, placenta, and kidney
- Increase is normal in pregnancy
- Increased in biliary obstruction, bone metastasis or destruction, and malignant liver tumors

Benign transient hyperphosphatemia can occur in young children for 4–8 weeks.

Amylase

Newborn	0–44 U/L
Adult	0–88 U/L

- Major sources: pancreas, salivary glands, and ovaries
- Most common reason for increase is pancreatitis
- Levels are high in alcoholism, pregnancy, and diabetic ketoacidosis with a salivary origin

Antinuclear Antibodies (ANAs)

Not significant	<1:80
Likely significant	>1:320

- Used to rule out systemic lupus erythematosus (SLE), but can also be increased in rheumatoid arthritis (RA), scleroderma, carcinoma, tuberculosis (TB), and hepatitis

Antistreptolysin-O (ASO) Titer

Preschool	<1:85
School age	<1:170
Older adult	<1:85

- A 4x rise in paired serial specimens is significant
- Antibodies appear 7–10 days after acute streptococcal infection
- Also can be increased in liver disease

Aspartate Aminotransferase (AST)/Serum Glutamic-oxaloacetic Transaminase (SGOT)

Newborn/infant	20–65 U/L
Child/adult	0–35 U/L

- Major sources: liver, skeletal muscle, kidney, myocardium, and erythrocytes
- Increased in liver necrosis, Reye's syndrome, hepatitis, myocardial infarction (MI), and infectious mononucleosis
- Not likely to be decreased

Bicarbonate (HCO_3)

Infant	20–24 mEq/L
>2 years	22–26 mEq/L

- Functions as a buffer to keep pH normal
- Increased in metabolic alkalosis
- Decreased in metabolic acidosis

Bilirubin (Total)

Term infants	
Cord	<2 mg/dL
0–1 day	<6 mg/dL
1–2 days	<8 mg/dL
3–7 days	<12 mg/dL
>1 month	0.2–1 mg/dL
Adult	0.1–1 mg/dL

Direct (Bili conjugated [BC])

0–0.4 mg/dL

BC is increased in conditions that cause obstruction in normal bile flow.

Indirect (Bili unconjugated [BU])

Total − direct = indirect
(Total − BC = BU)

BU is increased in any condition that causes hemolysis of red blood cells (RBCs).

Blood Urea Nitrogen (BUN)

5–25 mg/dL

- Used primarily to assess renal function but is affected by protein breakdown, hydration, and liver failure

- Increased in severe dehydration and impaired renal perfusion
- Decreased in overhydration

Calcium-Total Serum (Ca)

<1 week	7–12 mg/dL
Child	8–10.5 mg/dL
Adult	8.5–10.5 mg/dL

- Increased in dehydration, vitamin D intoxication, and metastatic bone disease
- Decreased in chronic renal disease, severe malnutrition, and low albumin levels

Chloride (Cl)

94–106 mEq/L

- Increases as sodium increases
- Decreases commonly caused by loss from vomiting, diarrhea, and diuretics

Cholesterol

Infant	53–135 mg/dL
Child	70–175 mg/dL
Adolescent	120–210 mg/dL
Adult	140–250 mg/dL

>35 mg/dL (high-density lipoprotein) "good cholesterol"
<110 mg/dL (low-density lipoprotein) "bad cholesterol"

- Increased in those with diets high in cholesterol and saturated fats
- Some also have genetic predispositions
- Decreased in hyperthyroidism, severe liver damage, and malnutrition

Carbon Dioxide Content (CO_2)

Infant/child	20–24 mEq/L
Adult	24–30 mEq/L

- Is an indirect measure of serum bicarbonate and is usually 2 mEq/L greater than the actual bicarbonate level
- Changes signify changes in acid-base balance

Complete Blood Count (CBC)

RBCs

Newborn	5.5–6 million/mm^3
Child	4.6–4.8 million/mm^3

Adult	(male)	4.6–5.9 million/mm^3
	(female)	4.2–5.4 million/mm^3

- Increased number in high altitudes, increased physical strain, chronic lung disease, and cyanotic heart disease
- Decreased because of abnormal loss or destruction and bone marrow suppression

Descriptors of RBCs

Hypochromic—less color
Normochromic—normal color
Microcytic—small size
Normocytic—normal size
Macrocytic—large size

Hemoglobin (Hgb, Hb)

Newborn		17–19 g
Child		14–17 g
Adult	(male)	13–18 g
	(female)	12–16 g

- If increased, look at in relation to the number and size of RBCs
- Decreased in all conditions that cause a decrease in RBCs (e.g., abnormal [Hgb], increased fragility leading to increased destruction)

Hematocrit (Hct)

Newborn		up to 65%
Child (mean)		
2 weeks		53%
1 month		44%
2 months		35%
6 months–2 years		36%
2–6 years		37%
6–12 years		40%
12–18 years	(male)	43%
	(female)	41%
Adult	(male)	45%–52%
	(female)	37%–48%

- Is the packed cell volume or the percentage of RBCs in plasma
- Is roughly three times the Hgb
- Capillary values may be 5%–10% higher than vena puncture
- Increased in normally hydrated child indicates a true increase in RBCs
- Can be increased in dehydration and decreased in over hydration

Mean corpuscular volume (MCV)

Newborn	95–121 μm^3
6–24 months	70–86 μm^3

Gradually increases to 78–98 μm^3
Describes the average RBC volume

Hct ÷ RBC = MCV

- If less than 86 μm^3, the RBCs are considered microcytic and possibly indicates iron-deficiency anemia, lead poisoning, or thalassemia
- If greater than 98 μm^3, the RBCs are considered macrocytic and indicates possible pernicious anemia or folic-acid deficiency

Mean corpuscular hemoglobin (MCH)

27–32 pg

- Amount of Hgb in a single cell

Hgb ÷ RBC = MCH

Mean corpuscular hemoglobin concentration (MCHC)

32%–36%

- Proportion of each cell occupied by Hgb
- Increased in congenital spherocytosis
- May be increased in normal newborns and sickle cell disease
- Decreased in microcytic anemias including iron-deficiency anemia

RBC Distribution Width (RDW)

11.5%–14.5%

- Variation of cell width
- May help assess types of anemias
- Iron-deficiency anemia increases the RDW, thalassemia does not
- Also increased in anisocytosis, reticulocytosis, and hemolysis, as well as in newborns

Platelets (Plt)

Newborn	100,000–290,000/mm^3
Child	150,000–350,000/mm^3
Adult	150,000–350,000/mm^3

- Have an 8- to 10-day life span
- Aid in coagulation by adhering and clumping to the wall of the vessel

- Increased (thrombocytosis) in malignancy and polycythemia
- Decreased (thrombocytopenia) in idiopathic thrombocytopenic purpura (ITP), after viral illness, in AIDS, in bone marrow suppression, and in patients with enlarged spleens, which destroy them too quickly

White blood cells (WBCs)

Newborn	10,000–35,000
Child	8,000–14,500
Adult	4,300–10,000

- Total WBC count
- Increased in bacterial infection and leukemias, especially acute lymphocytic leukemia
- Decreased in bone marrow suppression, in overwhelming sepsis, and with certain types of chemotherapy

Differential (diff) (mean %)

	Neutophils	Bands	Lymphocytes	Monocytes	Eosinophils
Newborn	61	4	31	6	2
1 mo	35		56	7	3
6 mo	32		61	5	3
1 yr	31		61	5	3
2 yr	33		59	5	3
4 yr	42		50	5	3
6 yr	51		42	5	3
8 yr	53		39	4	2
10 yr	54		38	4	2
16 yr	57		35	5	3
21 yr	59		34	4	3

- Total percentage must add up to 100%
- Left shift is usually seen in bacterial infections
- The left side of the diff (neutophils and bands) increases
- Left shift also may be calculated as an immature to total (IT) neutrophil ratio of 0.20 or greater:
  IT = bands (immature) ÷ bands and neutrophils (total) ≥ 0.20

Absolute neutrophil count (ANC) = % of neutrophils + % of bands × number of WBCs

Example: WBC count = 10,000, neutrophils = 51% bands = 2%
51% + 2% = 53% 10,000 = ANC of 5,300

Neutropenia is an ANC < 1,500

- Segs: segmented neutrophils, mature form

- Bands: immature form of neutrophil
  - Are increased in bacterial infections, inflammatory processes, and tissue necrosis
  - Are decreased (neutropenia) in viral diseases, hepatitis, influenza, measles, mumps, rubella, and overwhelming infections
- Lymph: lymphocytes:
  - Principal component of the immune system:
    T lymphocyte is approximately 60%–80%
    B lymphocyte is approximately 5%–15%
    Non-T, non-B lymphocyte is approximately 10%–20%
  - Are increased in viral infections, mumps, hepatitis, retrovirus, infectious mononucleosis, tumors, and TB
  - Significantly increased in lymphocytic leukemias
  - Decreased in AIDS, severe malnutrition, and any condition that increases the neutrophils
- Mono: monocytes
  - Increase usually results from chronic conditions such as TB, malaria, and Rocky Mountain spotted fever
- Baso: basophils
  - Increased in malignancy
- Eos: eosinophils
  - Increased in allergic reactions, asthma, drug reactions, and parasitic infections
  - Decreased in corticosteroid use

Creatinine (Serum)

Newborn	0.3–1 mg/dL
Infant	0.2–0.4 mg/dL
Child	0.3–0.7 mg/dL
Adolescent	0.5–1 mg/dL
Adult (male)	0.6–1.3 mg/dL
(female)	0.5–1.2 mg/dL

- Used only to evaluate renal function
- Does not increase until at least half the nephrons are nonfunctioning

Erythrocyte Sedimentation Rate (ESR)

Newborn	0–4 mm/hr
Child	4–20 mm/hr
Adult (male)	0–20 mm/hr
(female)	0–10 mm/hr

- Normally increased during pregnancy
- Increase usually results from inflammation or tissue injury

- >100 mm/hr usually is a result of infection, malignant tumors, or collagen diseases
- Often used to monitor the course of RA, pelvic inflammatory disease, or infectious states in persons with AIDS

Ferritin

Newborn	25–200 ng/mL
1 mo	200–600 ng/mL
6 mo	50–200 ng/mL
6 mo–15 yr	7–140 ng/mL
Adult (male)	15–200 ng/mL
(female)	12–150 ng/mL

- Directly related to the amount of iron in storage
- Increased in chronic illness, malignancy, and chronic transfusions
- Decreased in malnutrition

Gamma-glutamyl Transferase (GGT)

0–3 wk	0–130 U/L
3 wk–3 mo	4–120 U/L
>3 mo (male)	5–65 U/L
(female)	5–35 U/L
1–15 yr	0–23 U/L
Adult (male)	11–50 U/L
(female)	7–32 U/L

- Major sources: liver, kidney, prostate, and spleen
- Increased in biliary obstruction, malignant tumor, and alcohol abuse

Glucose

Term	40–110 mg/dL
1 wk–16 yr	60–105 mg/dL
Adult	70–110 mg/dL

- Most common reason for persistent increase is diabetes mellitus
  - Mild diabetic acidosis 300–450 mg/dL
  - Moderate diabetic acidosis 450–600 mg/dL
  - Severe diabetic acidosis ≥600 mg/dL
  - Decreased with too little food intake and increased exercise
  - Spills into the urine when blood glucose ranges from 160–190 mg/dL

Hemoglobin A_{1c}

All ages 5%–7.5%

- Indication of blood sugar control over time

Iron (Serum)

Newborn		100–250 μg/dL
Infant		40–100 μg/dL
Child		50–120 μg/dL
Adolescent	(male)	50–160 μg/dL
	(female)	40–150 μg/dL
Adult		50–150 μg/dL (male slightly increased)

- Evening levels are lower, so draw in morning
- Should have no iron supplements for 24 hours before test
- Decreased in iron-deficiency anemia

Lead (Pb)

Class		
I	≤ 9 μg/dL	Low risk; retest at 2 years of age
IIA	10–14 μg/dL	Borderline: retest every 3–4 months until three results are <15 μg/dL, then test annually
IIB	15–19 μg/dL	Retest every 2 months
III	20–44 μg/dL	Need medical evaluation; test for iron-deficiency anemia; environmental sources need to be identified and eliminated; may need pharmacologic treatment
IV	45–69 μg/dL	Need medical treatment, environmental assessment, and remediation within 48 hours
V	≥ 70 μg/dL	Need medical treatment, environmental assessment, and remediation immediately

(Siberry & Iannone, 2000.)

Fingerstick lead levels that are elevated need to be reconfirmed by venipuncture.

Magnesium

1.5–2 mEq/L

- Increased in renal failure and in patients receiving intravenous (IV) magnesium sulfate
- Decreased in chronic malnutrition, chronic aminoglycoside use, and chronic hypercalcemia

Phosphorus

Newborn	4.2–9.5 mg/dL
Infant	4.5–6.5 mg/dL
Child	3.5–6 mg/dL
Adult	2.7–4.5 mg/dL

- Increased in renal failure and vitamin D toxicity
- Decreased in malabsorption
- Most frequent and dangerous electrolyte disorder in hyperalimentation

Potassium (K)

<10 days	4.0–6.0 mEq/L
>10 days	3.5–5.0 mEq/L

- Increased in patients with inadequate renal output
- Decreased in patients with loss through the gastrointestinal (GI) tract from vomiting and nasogastric (NG) tube drainage
- Small changes have a great effect on cardiac muscle
- Hemolysis from squeezing finger or heel can falsely elevate results

Prealbumin

Newborn–6 wk	4–36 mg/dL
6 wk–16 yr	13–27 mg/dL
Adult	18–45 mg/dL

- Used to aid in nutritional assessment
- Decreased in malnutrition

Reticulocyte Count (Retic)

Newborn	3%–7%
1 mo	0.1%–1.7%
2–6 mo	0.7%–2.3%
2–18 yr	0.5%–1.0%
Adult (male)	0.8%–2.5%
(female)	0.8%–4.1%

- Are less mature RBCs
- Measure bone marrow function
- Increases result from increased destruction and the need for more RBCs from hemolysis of ABO incompatibility and sickle cell disease, or from increased loss from acute blood loss
- Will increase after treatment for iron-deficiency anemia is begun
- Decreased in abnormal bone marrow function

Sodium (Na)

135–145 mEq/L

- Changes not commonly seen because its concentration is always correlated with fluid balance

- Elevated in hypertonic dehydration with loss of large amounts of water without proportional losses of sodium
- Decreased in water intoxication in which loss of sodium and water is replaced with water only

Triglycerides (Fasting)

Age	Male (mg/dL)	Female (mg/dL)
0–5 yr	30–86	32–99
6–11 yr	31–108	35–114
12–15 yr	36–138	41–138
16–19 yr	40–163	40–128
20–29 yr	44–185	40–128
Over 29 yr	40–160	35–135

- Increased in nephrotic syndrome, hypothyroidism, and diabetes
- Decreased is rarely a problem

Uric Acid (Serum)

0–2 yr	2.4–4.6 mg/dL
2–12 yr	2.4–5.9 mg/dL
12–14 yr	2.4–6.4 mg/dL
Adult (male)	3.5–7.2 mg/dL
(female)	2.4–6.4 mg/dL

- Increased in gout, renal impairment, eclampsia, neoplastic disease, chemotherapy, radiation, and chronic malnutrition
- Decreased in syndrome of inappropriate antidiuretic hormone (SIADH), renal tubular defects, and liver disease

Urinalysis (UA)

Color	Light yellow to dark amber
Clarity	Should be clear
Odor	Fresh specimen should not have ammonia odor
PH	4.3–8, average 6; is affected by diet; most bacteria (except *Escherichia* coli) increase the pH, creating alkaline urine
Specific gravity (sp. gr.)	Infants–2 years 1.001–1.018 Adults 1.001–1.040 (usually 1.015–1.025) If fixed at 1.010 (sp. gr. of plasma), the kidney has lost the ability to concentrate urine The higher the number, the more concentrated the urine

Protein	Usually negative; persistent proteinuria is indicative of renal dysfunction
Sugar	Usually negative; if positive, blood glucose is at least 160 mg/dL
Ketone	Negative; if positive, body is burning fat for energy
Nitrites and leukocyte esterase (LE)	Should be negative; if positive, usually has a urinary tract infection (UTI)
Bilirubin	Negative; if positive, is the first indication of liver disease before jaundice
Urobilinogen	Increased in hemolytic disease
Sediment	Crystals—Uric acid, calcium oxalate, and triple phosphates are normal Casts—Most are pathologic; a few hyaline casts are normal; WBC casts (>4–5) are associated with infection; RBC casts are associated with damage to the glomerular membrane

Zinc

70–150 μg/dL

- Major sources: liver and organs, muscles, bones, RBCs, and WBCs
- Increased in copper deficiency
- Decreased in iron-deficiency anemia

CONVERSION TABLES FOR COMMONLY USED APPROXIMATE EQUIVALENTS

1 gram (g)	=	1,000 milligrams (mg)
1 g	=	1 cubic centimeter (cc)
1 g	=	15 or 16 grains (gr)
60 or 65 mg	=	1 gr
1 mg	=	1,000 micrograms (μg)
1 kilogram (kg)	=	1,000 g
1 kg	=	2.2 pounds
1 milliliter (mL)	=	1 cc
1 mL	=	15 or 16 minims
1 drop (gtt.)	=	1 minim
4 mL	=	1 dram (fluid dram)
5 mL	=	1 teaspoon (tsp)

15 mL	=	1 tablespoon (Tbsp)
30 mL	=	1 ounce (fluid ounce) (oz)
500 mL	=	1 pint (pt)
1,000 mL	=	1 liter (L)
1 L	=	1 quart (qt)
1 inch (in.)	=	2.54 centimeters (cm)
1 cm	=	10 millimeters (mm)

For quick *rough* conversions without using a calculator:

Pounds to kg: Subtract the first number in the pounds (or first 2 numbers if weight is greater than 100) from the total pounds and divide by 2.

Example: Weight = 45 pounds
$45 - 4 = 41$
$41 \div 2 = 20.5$ kg (rough conversion) vs.
$45 \div 2.2 = 20.45$ (calculator result)
Weight = 132 pounds
$132 - 13 = 119$
$119 \div 2 = 59.5$ kg (rough conversion) vs.
$132 \div 2.2 = 60$ (calculator result)

ABBREVIATIONS COMMONLY USED IN PEDIATRIC NURSING

ABD	abdominal
ABG	arterial blood gas
ACE	angiotensin-converting enzyme
ACTH	adrenocorticotropic hormone
ADD/ADHD	attention deficit disorder/attention deficit hyperactivity disorder
AFB	acid-fast bacillus
AGN	acute glomerulonephritis
$AgNO_3$	silver nitrate
AIDS	acquired immune deficiency syndrome
ALT	alanine aminotransferase (SGPT)
ALTE	apparent life-threatening event
ANA	antinuclear antibody
ANC	absolute neutrophil count
AOM	acute otitis media
AP	anteroposterior
AS	aortic stenosis
ASA	acetylsalicylic acid
ASD	atrial septal defect

ASO	antistreptolysin-O
AST	aspartate aminotransferase (SGOT)
A-V	atrioventricular
AV	arteriovenous
AZT	zidovudine
BAL	dimercaprol
BC	blood culture
BCS	battered child syndrome
b.i.d.	two times per day
BiPAP	bilevel positive airway pressure
BM	bowel movement
BP	blood pressure
BPD	bronchopulmonary dysplasia
bpm	beats per minute
BRATS	bananas, rice, applesauce, toast, saltines
BUN	blood urea nitrogen
Ca	calcium
calcium EDTA	calcium disodium edetate
CAT	computerized axial tomography
CBC	complete blood count
cc	cubic centimeter
CCB	calcium channel blocker
CDC	Centers for Disease Control and Prevention
CF	cystic fibrosis
CFU	colony-forming unit
CHD	congenital heart disease
	cyanotic heart disease
CHF	congestive heart failure
CL	central line
cm	centimeter
CMV	cytomegalovirus
CNS	central nervous system
CO	carbon monoxide
CO_2	carbon dioxide
CoA	coarctation of aorta
CP	cerebral palsy
CPAP	continuous positive airway pressure
CPK	creatinine phosphokinase
CPR	cardiopulmonary resuscitation
Cr	creatinine
C&S	culture and sensitivity
CSF	cerebrospinal fluid

C-spine	cervical spine
CT	computed tomography
CVA	costovertebral angle
CVL	central venous line
c/w	compared with
CXR	chest x-ray
dc	discharge
D/C	discontinue
DDAVP	desmopressin
DDH	developmental dysplasia of the hip
DEA	Drug Enforcement Agency
DIC	disseminated intravascular coagulation
diff	differential
DKA	diabetic ketoacidosis
dl or dL	deciliter
DNA	deoxyribonucleic acid
DNR	do not resuscitate
DOB	date of birth
DTaP	diphtheria-tetanus-acellular pertussis (vaccine)
DTP	diphtheria-tetanus-pertussis (vaccine)
DTR	deep tendon reflex
D_5W	5% dextrose in water
$D_{25}W$	25% dextrose in water
Dx	diagnosis
EBV	Epstein-Barr virus
ECD	endocardial cushion defect
ECG/EKG	electrocardiogram
ECHO	echocardiogram
ED	emergency department
EDTA	ethylenediaminetetraacetic acid
EEG	electroencephalogram
ELISA	enzyme-linked immunosorbent assay
EM	erythema multiforme
ENT	ear, nose, and throat
EOM	extraocular movement
EOS	eosinophil
ESR	erythrocyte sedimentation rate
ET	endotracheal
ETT	endotracheal tube
FB	foreign body
FDA	Food and Drug Administration
Fe	iron

FEV_1	forced expiratory volume in one second
FH_X	family history
FOC	formula of choice
	frontal occipital circumference
FSH	follicle-stimulating hormone
FTT	failure to thrive
F/U	follow-up
FUO	fever of unknown origin
F_X	fracture
g	gram
GABHS	group A beta hemolytic streptococcus
GC	gonococcal
G-CSF	granulocyte colony-stimulating factor
GE	gastroenteritis
GI	gastrointestinal
GnRH	gonadotropin-releasing hormone
gtt.	drops
GTT	glucose tolerance test
	glutamyl transferase
GU	genitourinary
GYN	gynecology
HA	headache
HbA_{1c}	glycosylated hemoglobin
HbCV	*Haemophilus influenzae* type b conjugate vaccine
HBIG	hepatitis B immune globulin
HBsAg	hepatitis B surface antigen
HBV	hepatitis B virus
HC	head circumference
hCG	human chorionic gonadotropin
HCO_3	bicarbonate
Hct	hematocrit
HDL	high-density lipoprotein
HEENT	head, eyes, ears, nose, and throat
Hg	mercury
Hgb	hemoglobin
HIB	*Haemophilus influenzae* type b (vaccine)
HIV	human immunodeficiency virus
H/O	history of
H_2O_2	hydrogen peroxide
H&P	history and physical
HPV	human papillomavirus
HR	heart rate

h.s.	at bedtime
HSP	Henoch-Schönlein purpura
HSV	herpes simplex virus
HTN	hypertension
HUS	hemolytic uremic syndrome
H_x	history
IBD	inflammatory bowel disease
ICP	intracranial pressure
ICS	intercostal space
I&D	incision and drainage
IDDM	insulin-dependent diabetes mellitus
IDM	infant of a diabetic mother
IgA	immunoglobulin A
IgG	immunoglobulin G
IgM	immunoglobulin M
IID	intermittent infusion device
IM	intramuscular
INH	isoniazid
IO	intraosseus
I&O	intake and output
IPV	inactivated polio vaccine
ITP	immune thrombocytopenic purpura
IUD	intrauterine device
IUGR	intrauterine growth retardation
IV	intravenous
IVIG	intravenous immune globulin
IVP	intravenous pyelogram
JDM	juvenile diabetes mellitus
JRA	juvenile rheumatoid arthritis
K	potassium
Kcal	kilocalorie
KCl	potassium chloride
KD	Kawasaki disease
kg	kilogram
KOH	potassium hydroxide
LDL	low-density lipoprotein
LET	lidocaine, epinephrine, tetracaine
LFTs	liver function tests
LH	luteinizing hormone
LIP	lymphoid interstitial pneumonitis
LP	lumbar puncture
LTB	laryngotracheobronchitis

LUQ	left upper quadrant
max	maximum
MCHC	mean corpuscular hemoglobin concentration
MCL	midclavicular line
MCV	mean corpuscular volume
MDI	metered-dose inhaler
mEq	milliequivalent
mg	milligram
min	minute
ml or mL	milliliter
mm	millimeter
MMR	measles-mumps-rubella (vaccine)
MR	mental retardation
MRI	magnetic resonance imaging
MSBP	Munchausen syndrome by proxy
Na	sodium
$NaHCO_3$	sodium bicarbonate
NEC	necrotizing enterocolitis
NF	neurofibromatosis
NG	nasogastric
NH_3	ammonia
NIDDM	non–insulin-dependent diabetes mellitus
NP	nasopharyngeal
NPO	nothing by mouth
NSAID	nonsteroidal anti-inflammatory drug
O_2	oxygen
OCD	obsessive-compulsive disorder
OD	right eye
OM	otitis media
OPV	oral polio vaccine
OS	left eye
OTC	over the counter
OU	each eye
oz	ounce
P	phosphorus
Pb	lead
PBS	phenobarbital sodium
PCA	patient-controlled analgesia
pCO_2	partial pressure of carbon dioxide
PCP	*Pneumocystis carinii* pneumonia
PDA	patent ductus arteriosus

PE	physical examination
PEF	peak expiratory flow
PEFR	peak expiratory flow rate
PET	positron emission tomography
PFM	peak flow meter
PGG	pH, glucose, guaiac
PID	pelvic inflammatory disease
PKU	phenylketonuria
PMI	point of maximal impulse
PNET	primitive neuroectodermal tumor
PO	by mouth
Po_2	partial pressure of oxygen
PO_4	phosphate
PPD	purified protein derivative (used in tuberculosis skin test)
PPS	post–pericardial syndrome
p.r.n.	as needed
pt	patient
PT	prothrombin time
PTSD	post-traumatic stress disorder
PTT	partial thromboplastin time
PUD	peptic ulcer disease
PVC	premature ventricular contraction
q	every
q.d.	one time per day
q.i.d.	four times per day
q.o.d.	every other day
RA	rheumatoid arthritis
RAD	reactive airway disease
RBC	red blood cell
RDS	respiratory distress syndrome
REM	rapid eye movement
RF	rheumatic fever
RMSF	Rocky Mountain spotted fever
R/O	rule out
ROM	range of motion
ROS	rule out sepsis
RR	respiratory rate
RSV	respiratory syncytial virus
RUQ	right upper quadrant
R_X	prescription

SaO_2	oxygen saturation
SB	spina bivida
	sternal border
SBE	subacute bacterial endocarditis
SCC	sickle cell crisis
SCD	sickle cell disease
SCFE	slipped capital femoral epiphysis
SIADH	syndrome of inappropriate antidiuretic hormone
SIDS	sudden infant death syndrome
sig.	directions
SLE	systemic lupus erythematosus
SO	significant other
SOB	shortness of breath
SOM	serous otitis media
S/P	status post
sp. gr.	specific gravity
STD	sexually transmitted disease
S_X	symptoms
T	temperature
T_3	triiodothyronine
T_4	tetraiodothyronine
T&A	tonsillectomy and adenoidectomy
TAC	tetracaine, adrenalin (epinephrine), and cocaine
TB	tuberculosis
TEF	tracheoesophageal fistula
TGA	transposition of the great arteries
TGV	transposition of the great vessels
t.i.d.	three times per day
TM	tympanic membrane
TOF	tetralogy of Fallot
TORCH	toxoplasmosis, other infections, rubella, cytomegalovirus, and herpes simplex
TPA	total parenteral alimentation
TPN	total parenteral nutrition
TRH	thyroid-releasing hormone
TSH	thyroid-stimulating hormone
tsp	teaspoon
T_X	treatment
U	unit
UA	urinalysis
URI	upper respiratory infection
US	ultrasound

UTI	urinary tract infection
VCUG	voiding cystourethrogram
VP	ventriculoperitoneal
vs	versus
VS	vital signs
VSD	ventricular septal defect
WBC	white blood cell
WHO	World Health Organization
w/u	work-up

WEST NOMOGRAM

Place a straight edge from the patient's height in the left column to his or her weight in the right column. The point of intersection on the body surface area (BSA) column indicates the BSA.

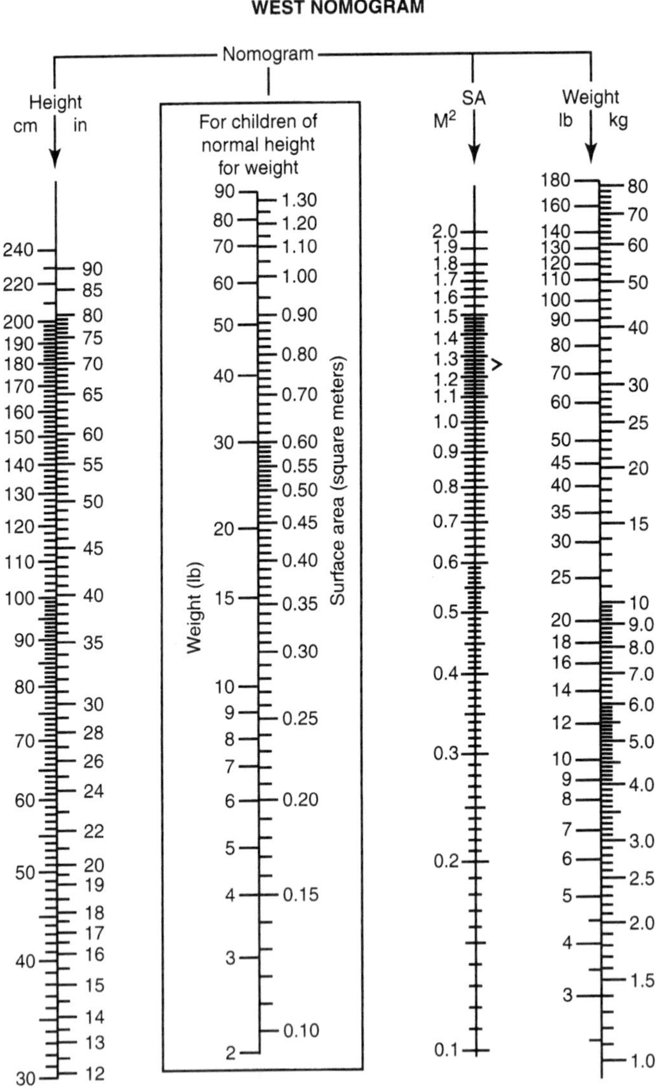

From *Nelson Textbook of Pediatrics* (15th ed.) by R.E. Behrman, R.M. Kleigman, & A.M. Arvin, 1996, Philadelphia: Saunders. Reprinted with permission.

CHAPTER 4

DRUG ADMINISTRATION

COMMON PEDIATRIC DRUGS

Efforts have been made to ensure that drug dosage information herein is accurate and reflects acceptable standards at the time of publication. However, changes in practice continually occur. Therefore, readers are advised to check product information included with each drug to be sure that changes have not been made.

acetaminophen (Tylenol and others)

Indications

(analgesic; antipyretic)
Mild to moderate pain, fever.

Administration

10–15 mg/kg/dose q4–6h; 5 doses in 24 hr (max. dose: 4 g/24 hr, 5 doses/24 hr)

Dosing by age:	PO or PR
0–3 mo:	40 mg/dose
4–11 mo:	80 mg/dose
12–24 mo:	120 mg/dose
2–3 yr:	160 mg/dose
4–5 yr:	240 mg/dose
6–8 yr:	320 mg/dose
9–10 yr:	400 mg/dose
11–12 yr:	480 mg/dose
Adult:	325–650 mg/dose

Nursing Implications

Dose standardization common. Contraindicated in known glucose-6-phosphate dehydrogenase (G6PD) deficiency. Rectal absorption variable. Use cautiously in severe hepatic disease. Administer with food to decrease gastrointestinal (GI) upset. Assess and document effect 30–60 min after administration. Can cause rash, blood dyscrasias.

acyclovir (Zovirax)

Indications

(antiviral agent)

Used in treatment of herpes simplex virus (HSV) and varicella-zoster virus in healthy, nonpregnant ≥13 yr olds. Also used in children ≥12 mo with immune or chronic disorders.

Administration

HSV:

Initial infection:

IV: 15 mg/kg/24 hr ÷ q8h × 5–7 days

PO: 1,200 mg/24 hr ÷ q8h × 7–10 days

Recurrence:

PO: 1,200 mg/24 hr ÷ q8h *or* 1,600 mg/24 hr ÷ q12h × 5 days

Neonatal HSV and HSV encephalitis:

All ages: 30 mg/kg/24 hr ÷ q8h IV × 14–21 days

Term infants can have higher doses of 45–60 mg/kg/24 hr ÷ q8h IV

Zoster:

IV: 30 mg/kg/24 hr ÷ q8h × 7–10 days

PO: 4,000 mg/24 hr ÷ 5x/24 hr × 5–7 days for patients ≥12 yr

Varicella:

IV: 30 mg/kg/24 hr ÷ q8h × 7–10 days

PO: 80 mg/kg/24 hr ÷ q.i.d. × 5 days (start within 24 hr of rash onset) (max. dose: 3,200 mg/24 hr)

(max. dose of oral acyclovir in children is 80 mg/kg/24 hr)

IV dilution:

max. concentration: 7–10 mg/mL

usual concentration: 10 mg/mL over 60 min

Compatibility: 5% dextrose in water (D_5W), normal saline (NS), lactated ringers (LR)

Nursing Implications

Adequate hydration and slow IV administration essential to prevent crystal formation in renal tubules. Dose reduction required in renal impairment. Side effects include headache (HA), lethargy, skin rash, nausea, vomiting, and bone marrow suppression.

albuterol (Proventil, Ventolin)

Indications

(β_2-adrenergic agent)

Bronchodilator used in asthma or reactive airway disease (RAD) for prevention and relief of bronchospasm.

Administration

PO:	
<6 yr:	0.3 mg/kg/24 hr ÷ q8h (max. dose: 12 mg/24 hr)
6–11 yr:	6 mg/24 hr ÷ t.i.d. (max. dose: 24 mg/24 hr)
≥12 yr/adult:	2–4 mg dose t.i.d.–q.i.d. (max. dose: 32 mg/24 hr)
Inhalations:	
Aerosol (metered-dose inhaler [MDI]):	1–2 puffs (90–180 μg) q4–6h p.r.n.
Nebulized:	
<1 yr:	0.05–0.15 mg/kg/dose q4–6h
1–5 yr:	1.25–2.5 mg/dose q4–6h
5–12 yr:	2.5 mg/dose q6h
>12 yr:	2.5–5 mg/dose q6h

Higher doses can be used in acute exacerbations.

Nursing Implications

Administer PO with meals to decrease gastric irritation. Use spacer with MDI to enhance efficacy. Side effects include tachycardia, palpitations, tremor, insomnia, nervousness, nausea, and HA. Side effects more pronounced with PO doses, less with nebulizer, and least with MDI.

allopurinol (Zyloprim and others)

Indications

(uric acid lowering agent; xanthine oxidase inhibitor)

Used to prevent attacks of gouty arthritis and nephropathy. Also used to treat secondary hyperuricemia and for prevention of recurrent calcium oxalate calculi.

Administration

Child:	10 mg/kg/24 hr ÷ b.i.d.–q.i.d. PO (max. dose: 800 mg/24 hr)
Adult:	200–300 mg/24 hr ÷ b.i.d.–t.i.d. PO

Nursing Implications

Side effects include rash, neuritis, hepatotoxicity, GI disturbances, bone marrow suppression, and drowsiness.

amikacin (Amikin)

Indications

(antibiotic; aminoglycoside)

Used in treatment of serious gram-negative bacillary infections and staphylococcal infections when penicillin and other less toxic drugs are contraindicated.

Administration

Infant/child: 15–22.5 mg/kg/24 hr ÷ q8h IV/IM

Adult: 15 mg/kg/24 hr ÷ q8–12h IV/IM (max. dose: 1.5 g/24 hr, then monitor levels)

IV dilution: 5 mg/mL over 30–60 min; 50 mg/mL central venous line (CVL)

Compatibility: D_5W, NS, LR

Nursing Implications

Therapeutic levels must be monitored. Peak: 20–30 mg/L; trough: 5–10 mg/L. Dose adjusted in renal insufficiency. Patient needs to be well hydrated. May cause ototoxicity, nephrotoxicity, neuromuscular blockade, and rash.

amiodarone hydrochloride (Cordarone)

Indications

(antiarrhythmic agent, class III)

Used to manage resistant, life-threatening ventricular arrhythmias unresponsive to conventional treatment with less toxic agents.

Administration

Child PO:

<1 yr: 600–800 mg/1.73m²/24 hr ÷ q12–24h, then decrease to 200–400 mg/1.73m²/24 hr

≥1 yr: 10–15 mg/kg/24 hr ÷ q12–24h × 4–14 days or until adequate control is achieved, then decrease to 5 mg/kg/24 hr ÷ q12–24h

Child IV: (limited data available) 5 mg/kg over 30 min followed by a continuous infusion starting at 5μg/kg/min; may be increased to a max. dose of 10μg/kg/min *or* 20 mg/kg/24 hr

IV dilution: 2 mg/mL *or* 6 mg/mL CVL

Compatibility: D_5W

Nursing Implications

Proposed therapeutic levels with chronic oral use is 1–2.5 mg/L. Side effects include asymptomatic corneal microdeposits, altered liver enzymes, paresthesias, ataxia, tremor, and hyperthyroidism or hypothyroidism.

amitriptyline (Elavil, Emitrip, Endep, Enovil)

Indications

(tricyclic antidepressant; antimigraine agent)

Used to treat various forms of depression, as an analgesic for certain chronic and neuropathic pain, and as a migraine prophylaxis.

Administration

Chronic pain management:

- Child: Initially 0.1 mg/kg q.h.s. PO; may increase over 2–3 wk to 0.5–2 mg/kg q.h.s. PO

Antidepressant:

- Child: 1 mg/kg/24 hr ÷ t.i.d. PO × 3 days, then increase to 1.5 mg/kg/24 hr (max. dose: 5 mg/kg/24 hr)
- Adolescent: 10 mg t.i.d. with 20 mg q.h.s. PO (max. dose: 200 mg/24 hr)
- Adult: 40–100 mg/24 hr q.h.s.–b.i.d. PO (max. dose: 300 mg/24 hr
  20–30 mg q.i.d. IM (convert to PO as soon as possible)

Nursing Implications

Monitor electrocardiogram (ECG), blood pressure (BP), and heart rate (HR) for doses >3 mg/kg/24 hr. Maximum antidepressant effect takes 2 wk. Therapeutic level is 100–250 ng/mL and is checked 8 hr after PO dose and after 4–5 days of continuous dosing. Side effects include sedation, urinary retention, constipation, dry mouth, dizziness, drowsiness, and arrhythmia. Do not give IV. May administer with food to decrease GI upset.

amoxicillin (Amoxil, Trimox, Wymox, Polymox)

Indications

(antibiotic; aminopenicillin)

Used in treatment of a variety of infections including, most commonly, otitis media (OM), as a first-line drug. Also used in sinusitis, respiratory and genitourinary (GU) tract infections, and for subacute bacterial endocarditis (SBE) prophylaxis.

Administration

Child: 20–50 mg/kg/24 hr ÷ q8h PO of 125- or 250-mg/5 cc strength *or* 25–45 mg/kg/24 hr ÷ b.i.d. PO of 200- or 400-mg/5 cc strength

Higher doses of 75–90 mg/kg/24 hr ÷ t.i.d. have been recommended for treatment of resistant *Streptococcus pneumoniae* in OM.

Adult: 250–500 mg/dose q8h PO (max. dose: 2–3 g/24 hr)

Endocarditis prophylaxis: 50 mg/kg 1 hr before procedure (not to exceed adult dose)

Nursing Implications

Most common side effects are rashes and diarrhea. Food does not interfere with absorption.

amoxicillin/clavulanate (Augmentin)

Indications

(antibiotic; aminopenicillin with β-lactamase inhibitor)

Same as amoxicillin but extends its activity to include β-lactamase–producing strains of *Haemophilus influenzae* and *Branhamella (Neisseria) catarrhalis*.

Administration

Child <3 mo: 30 mg/kg/24 hr ÷ b.i.d. PO using 125-mg/5 cc strength

Child ≥3 mo, <40 kg: 20–40 mg/kg/24 hr ÷ t.i.d. PO of 125- or 250-mg/5 cc strength *or*
25–45 mg/kg/24 hr ÷ b.i.d. PO of 200- or 400-mg/5 cc strength

Adult: 250–500 mg/dose q8h PO *or* 875 mg q12h PO (max. dose: 2g/24 hr)

Nursing Implications

Incidence of diarrhea higher than with amoxicillin, but lower with b.i.d. dosing strength and schedule. Give with meals to help decrease GI side effects.

amphotericin B (Fungizone, Amphocin)

Indications

(antifungal)

Used in treatment of severe systemic infections and meningitis caused by susceptible fungi.

Administer

Topical: Apply b.i.d.–t.i.d.
PO: 100 mg q.i.d. for oral candidiasis
IV:
Test dose: 0.1 mg/kg/dose up to max. of 1 mg (followed by remaining initial dose)
Initial dose: 0.25–0.5 mg/kg/24 hr
Increment: Increase as tolerated by 0.25–0.5 mg/kg/24 hr q.d. or q.o.d.
Maintenance: 0.25–1 mg/kg/24 hr *or* 1.5 mg/kg/dose q.o.d. (max. dose: 1.5 mg/kg/24 hr)
IV dilution: Mix to concentration of 0.1 mg/mL (peripheral) *or* 0.2 mg/mL (CVL) over 2–6 hr
Compatibility: D_5W, $D_{10}W$, $D_{20}W$

Nursing Implications

Common infusion-related reactions are fever, chills, HA, hypotension, nausea, and vomiting. May need to premedicate with acetaminophen and diphenhydramine HCI (Benadryl) 30 min before and 4 hr after infusion.

ampicillin (Omnipen, Polycillin, Principen, Totacillin-N)

Indications

(antibiotic; aminopenicillin)

Used for treatment of OM, sinusitis, respiratory tract infections, GU infections, meningitis, septicemia, and suspected group B streptococcal infections as well as for endocarditis prophylaxis.

Administration

Neonate:
<7days, <2 kg: 50–100 mg/kg/24 hr ÷ q12h IV/IM
<7 days, ≥2 kg: 75–150 mg/kg/24 hr ÷ q8h IV/IM
≥7 days, <1.2 kg: 50–100 mg/kg/24 hr ÷ q12h IV/IM
≥7 days, 1.2–2 kg: 75–150 mg/kg/24 hr ÷ q8h IV/IM
≥7 days, > 2 kg: 100–200 mg/kg/24 hr ÷ q6h IV/IM
Child:
Mild to moderate infections: 100–200 mg/kg/24 hr ÷ q6h IV/IM
50–100 mg/kg/24 hr ÷ q6h PO (max. PO dose: 2–3g/24 hr)
Severe infections: 200–400 mg/kg/24 hr ÷ q4–6h IV/IM (max. IV/IM dose: 12g/24 hr)

Adult:	500–3,000 mg q4–6h IV/IM 250–500 mg q6h PO
IV dilution:	
Direct IV:	Up to 500 mg only, over 3–5 min >500 mg, over 10–15 min (max. concentration 100 mg/mL; not to exceed 100 mg/min)
Intermittent IV:	30 mg/mL over 15–30 min
Compatibility:	D_5W, NS preferred, LR, sterile water (SW)

Nursing Implications

Higher doses used to treat central nervous system (CNS) disease. Hypersensitivity rash commonly seen at 5–10 days. Administer PO dose with water on an empty stomach 1–2 hr before meals. Reconstituted ampicillin sodium effective for 1 hr after reconstitution. IV administration at >100 mg/min may cause seizures. Can also cause interstitial nephritis, diarrhea, and pseudomembranous enterocolitis.

ampicillin/sulbactam (Unasyn)

Indications

(antibiotic; aminopenicillin with β-lactamase inhibitor)

Used to treat susceptible bacterial infections involved with skin, abdominal, and gynecologic infections. Effective against β-lactamase–producing organisms.

Administration

(dosage based on ampicillin component)

Child:	
Mild to moderate infections:	100–200 mg/kg/24 hr ÷ q6h IV/IM
Severe infections:	200–400 mg/kg/24 hr ÷ q4–6h IV/IM
Adult:	1–2 g q6–8h IV/IM (max. dose: 8g ampicillin/24 hr)
IV dilution:	max. concentration 45 mg of Unasyn/mL over 10–15 min
Compatibility:	D_5W, NS

Nursing Implications

Dose adjusted in renal failure. Similar cerebrospinal fluid (CSF) distribution and side effects as ampicillin.

aspirin, acetylsalicylic acid, ASA (Anacin, Bayer, and others)

Indications

(nonsteroidal anti-inflammatory drug [NSAID]; antiplatelet agent; analgesic)

Mild pain and fever. Also useful as an antipyretic and in Kawasaki disease.

Administration

Analgesic/antipyretic:	10–15 mg/kg/dose q4h PO/PR up to a total of 60–80 mg/kg/24 hr (max. dose: 4g/24 hr)
Anti-inflammatory:	60–100 mg/kg/24 hr ÷ q6–8h PO
Kawasaki disease:	80–100 mg/kg/24 hr ÷ q.i.d. PO during febrile phase, then decrease to 3–5 mg/kg/24 hr q AM PO

Nursing Implications

Do not use in children <16 yr old with chickenpox or flu-like symptoms. Use with caution in GI disease. May cause GI upset, tinnitus, allergic reactions, liver toxicity, and platelet aggregation. Give with water, food, or milk to decrease GI upset. Therapeutic levels vary according to purpose of administration; consult laboratory.

azithromycin (Zithromax)

Indications

(antibiotic; macrolide)

Used to treat mild to moderate upper and lower respiratory infections, skin infections, acute OM, and sexually transmitted diseases (STDs).

Administration

Child:	
OM or community-acquired pneumonia (≥6 mo):	10 mg/kg on day 1 q.d. PO (max. dose: 500 mg), then 5 mg/kg on days 2–5 q.d. PO (max. dose: 250 mg)
Pharyngitis/tonsillitis (≥2 yr):	12 mg/kg/24 hr q.d. PO (max. dose: 500 mg/24 hr)
Adolescent/adult:	
Respiratory tract, skin, and soft tissue infection:	500 mg on day 1 q.d. PO, then 250 mg on days 2–5 q.d. PO
Acute pelvic inflammatory disease (PID):	500 mg q.d. IV × 1–2 days, then 250 mg q.d. PO to complete 7- to 10-day therapy
IV dilution:	1 mg/mL over 3 hr *or* 2 mg/mL over 1 hr. Do not infuse over a period <60 min.

Nursing Implications

Can cause increase in liver enzymes, cholestatic jaundice, and GI discomfort. Capsules and oral suspension should be administered on an empty stomach, 1 hr before or 2 hr after a meal. Tablets and oral powder (sachet) can be given with food.

beclomethasone dipropionate (Beclovent, Beconase, Beconase AQ, Vanceril, Vancenase, Vancenase AQ)

Indications

(corticosteroid)

Used as inhalation for long-term control of persistent bronchial asthma and intranasally for management of seasonal or perennial rhinitis and nasal polyposis.

Administration

Oral inhalation	
(42 μg/inhalation [puff]):	
6–12 yr:	1–2 puffs TID-QID *or* 2–4 puffs b.i.d. max. dose: 10 puffs/24 hr
>12 yr:	2 puffs t.i.d.–q.i.d. (max. dose: 12 puffs/24 hr)
Oral inhalation, double strength (84 μg/puff):	
6–12 yr:	2 puffs b.i.d. (max. dose: 5 puffs/24 hr)
>12 yr:	2 puffs b.i.d. (max. dose: 10 puffs/24 hr)
Nasal inhalation:	
6–12 yr:	1 spray each nostril t.i.d.
>12 yr:	1 spray each nostril b.i.d.–q.i.d. *or* 2 sprays each nostril b.i.d.
Aqueous nasal spray:	
>6 yr–adult:	1–2 sprays each nostril b.i.d.

Nursing Implications

Not recommended for use in children <6 yr. *Avoid* using higher-than-recommended doses because can cause hypothalamic, pituitary, or adrenal suppression. Onset for oral inhalation is 1–4 wk; for nasal inhalation it is a few days to 2 wk. If child objects to the taste, have him or her drink a glass of orange juice before inhaling. Shake nasal and oral inhalation containers well before using. Have child rinse mouth after oral inhalation to prevent thrush. Spacers recommended for oral inhalations to increase amount of medicine getting to lungs. Side effects include HA, sore throat, thrush, cough, sneezing, hoarseness, irritation and burning of the nasal mucosa, nasal ulceration, epistaxis, rhinorrhea, and nasal congestion.

bethanechol chloride (Urecholine)

Implications

(cholinergic agent)

Used in treatment of nonobstructive urinary retention and abdominal distension. Also effective in treatment of gastroesophageal (GE) reflux.

Administration

Child:

Abdominal distension/ urinary retention:	0.6 mg/kg/24 hr ÷ q6–8h PO 0.12–0.2 mg/kg/24 hr ÷ q6–8h SC
GE reflux:	0.1–0.2 mg/kg/dose ÷ q.i.d. (30 min a.c. and h.s.) PO (max. dose: 4 doses in 24 hr)
Adult:	10–50 mg q6–12h PO 2.5–5 mg t.i.d.–q.i.d. SC, up to 7.5–10 mg q4h SC for neurogenic bladder

Nursing Implications

Contraindicated in asthma, mechanical GI or GU obstruction, peptic ulcer disease, cardiac disease, hyperthyroidism, and seizure disorder. Can cause hypotension; nausea; abdominal cramps; and increased salivation, flushing, and bronchospasm. Administer on empty stomach to reduce nausea and vomiting. Do not give IM or IV.

bisacodyl (Dulcolax)

Indications

(laxative; stimulant)

Used to evacuate colon. Indicated in treatment of constipation associated with bed rest or spinal cord injury. Also used as preparation for surgery or X-ray studies.

Administration

PO:

Child:	0.3 mg/kg/24 hr *or* 5–10 mg 6 hr before desired effect
Adult (>12 yr):	5–15 mg q.d.

PR:

<2 yr:	5 mg
2–11 yr:	5–10 mg
>11 yr:	10 mg

Nursing Implications

Tablets should not be crushed or chewed. Do not give within 1 hr of milk or antacids. Can cause nausea and abdominal cramping. Oral dose effective in 6–10 hr. Rectal effective within 15–60 min.

calcitriol (Rocaltrol, Calcijex)

Indications

(active form of vitamin D, fat soluble)

Most potent form of vitamin D available. Used most often in management of hypocalcemia in chronic renal failure. Promotes absorption of calcium from GI tract.

Administration

Renal failure:

Child: Range 0.01–0.05 μg/kg/24 hr PO; is titrated in 0.005- to 0.01-μg/kg/24 hr increments q4–8wk based on clinical response
0.01–0.05 μg/kg/dose IV3x/wk

Adult: Initial dose 0.25 μg/dose PO with increment increase at 0.25 μg/dose PO q4–8wk
Usual dose 0.5–1 μg/24 hr
0.5 μg/24 hr IV given 3x/wk
Usual dose 0.5–3 μg/24 hr IV given 3x/wk

IV dilution: May be given undiluted as a bolus dose IV at the end of hemodialysis

Nursing Implications

Avoid using with antacids containing magnesium. Contraindicated in patients with hypercalcemia. Serum calcium and phosphorous levels must be monitored. Eating foods high in calcium can lead to hypercalcemia. Can cause weakness, HA, vomiting, constipation, and hypotonia. IV dosing used for patients undergoing hemodialysis.

captopril (Capoten)

Indications

(angiotensin-converting enzyme inhibitor; antihypertensive)

Used in management of hypertension. Also used in combination with other drugs for treatment of congestive heart failure (CHF).

Administration

Neonate: 0.1–0.4 mg/kg/24 hr q6–8h PO

Infant: Initial dose 0.15–0.3 mg/kg/dose PO titrated upward for desired effect (max. dose: 6 mg/kg/24 hr ÷ q.d.–q.i.d. PO)
Child: Initial dose 0.3–0.5 mg/kg/dose ÷ q8h PO titrated upward as needed (max. dose: 6 mg/kg/24 hr ÷ b.i.d.–q.i.d. PO)
Adolescent/adult: Initial dose 12.5–25 mg/dose b.i.d.–q.i.d. PO increased weekly by 25 mg/dose (max. dose: 450 mg/24 hr)

Nursing Implications

Administer on empty stomach 1 hr before or 2 hr after meals. Reaches peak 1–2 hr after administration. Check baseline BP before administration. Use of NSAIDs may result in reduced antihypertensive response to captopril. May cause rash, proteinuria, neutropenia, cough, angioedema, hyperkalemia, hypotension, and decreased taste perception with long-term use.

carbamazepine (Tegretol, Carbatrol)

Indications

(anticonvulsant)

Used to prevent tonic-clonic, mixed, and complex partial seizures. Also used to relieve pain in trigeminal neuralgia or diabetic neuropathy and for treatment of bipolar disorders.

Administration

Child:

<6 yr: Initial dose 10–20 mg/kg/24 hr ÷ b.i.d.–t.i.d. PO (q.i.d. for suspension)
Increase at increments q5–7 days up to 35 mg/kg/24 hr PO

6–12 yr: Initial dose 10 mg/kg/24 hr ÷ b.i.d. up to max. dose of 100 mg/dose b.i.d. PO
Increase 100 mg/24 hr at 1-wk intervals ÷ t.i.d.–q.i.d. until desired response
Maintenance dose: 20–30 mg/kg/24 hr ÷ b.i.d.–q.i.d. PO
Usual maintenance dose: 400–800 mg/24 hr (max. dose: 1,000 mg/24 hr)

>12 yr: Initial dose 200 mg b.i.d. PO
Increase 200 mg/24 hr at 1-wk intervals ÷ b.i.d.–q.i.d. until desired response
Maintenance dose: 800–1,200 mg/24 hr ÷ b.i.d.–q.i.d. PO (max. dose: 12–15 yr: 1,000 mg/24 hr; adult: 1.6–2.4 g/24 hr)

Nursing Implications

Contraindicated in patients taking monoamine oxidase (MAO) inhibitors. Therapeutic blood levels 4–12 mg/L. Monitoring of serum levels mandatory when patients are switched from any product to another. Erythromycin, isoniazid (INH), cimetidine, and verapamil increase carbamazepine levels. May cause decrease in activity of warfarin, doxycycline, oral contraceptives, cyclosporin, theophylline, phenytoin, benzodiazepines, ethosuximide, and valproic acid. Doses may be administered with food to decrease GI upset. Do not simultaneously administer oral suspension with other liquid medicines or diluents. Side effects include sedation, dizziness, diplopia, aplastic anemia, neutropenia, urinary retention, syndrome of inappropriate antidiuretic hormone (SIADH), and Stevens-Johnson syndrome. Check complete blood cell count (CBC) and liver function tests (LFTs) before course and monitor for hematologic and hepatic toxicity.

carbenicillin (Geocillin, Geopen, Pyopen)

Indications

(antibiotic; extended-spectrum penicillin)

Used in treatment of urinary tract infections (UTIs), asymptomatic bacteriuria, or prostatitis.

Administration

Mild infection:

Child:	30–50 mg/kg/24 hr ÷ q6h PO (max. dose: 2–3 g/24 hr)
Adult (UTI):	382–764 mg q6h PO

Nursing Implications

Use with caution in patients who are allergic to penicillin. Side effects include nausea, vomiting, diarrhea, abdominal cramps, and flatulence. May cause hepatotoxicity and furry tongue.

cefaclor (Ceclor)

Indications

(antibiotic; second-generation cephalosporin)

Used in treatment of OM; respiratory, skin, and bone and joint infections; and UTIs.

Administration

Infant/child: 20–40 mg/kg/24 hr ÷ q8h PO (max. dose: 2g/24 hr)
May give q12h in OM or pharyngitis

Adult: 250–500 mg/dose q8h PO (max. dose: 4g/24 hr)

Nursing Implications

Use with caution in children with penicillin sensitivity or impaired renal function. May cause a positive Coombs' test or a false-positive test for urinary glucose. Also can cause nausea, vomiting, diarrhea, and rash. Food or milk delays and decreases peak concentration with capsules and suspension, so give 1 hr before or 2 hr after meals.

cefazolin (Ancef, Kefzol)

Indications

(antibiotic; first-generation cephalosporin)

Used in treatment of serious skin infections; respiratory tract, urinary tract, and bone and joint infections; and septicemia. Also used as prophylactic antibiotic for invasive procedures.

Administration

Neonate:	
≤7 days:	40 mg/kg/24 hr ÷ q12h IV/IM
>7 days, ≤2 kg:	40 mg/kg/24 hr ÷ q12h IV/IM
>2 kg:	60 mg/kg/24 hr ÷ q8h IV/IM
Infant >1 mo/child:	50–100 mg/kg/24 hr ÷ q8h IV/IM (max. dose: 6g/24 hr)
Adult:	2–6g/24 hr ÷ q6–8h IV/IM (max. dose: 12g/24 hr)
IV dilution:	
Direct IV:	max. concentration: 100 mg/mL over 3–5 min.
Intermittent infusion:	20 mg/mL over 10–60 min.
Compatibility:	D_5W, NS, LR

Nursing Implications

Use with caution in children with penicillin sensitivity or impaired renal function. May cause phlebitis, leukopenia, thrombocytopenia, transient increase in liver enzymes, false-positive urine-reducing substance, and positive Coombs' test.

cefixime (Suprax)

Indications

(antibiotic; third-generation cephalosporin)

Used in treatment of mild UTIs, OM, bronchitis, pharyngitis, and tonsillitis.

Administration

Infant/child: 8 mg/kg/24 hr ÷ q12–24 hr PO (max. dose: 400 mg/24 hr)

Adolescent/adult: 400 mg/24 hr ÷ q12–24 hr PO

Nursing Implications

Use with caution in children with penicillin sensitivity or impaired renal function. Can cause diarrhea, abdominal pain, nausea, and HA. Administer with food to decrease GI upset. Tablets not effective in treatment of OM; use suspension.

cefotaxime (Claforan)

Indications

(antibiotic; third-generation cephalosporin)

Used in treatment of skin, bone, joint, urinary, gynecologic, respiratory, and intraabdominal infections, as well as septicemia and meningitis.

Administration

Neonate:	
≤7 days, <2 kg:	100 mg/kg/24 hr ÷ q12h IV/IM
≥2 kg:	100–150 mg/kg/24 hr ÷ q8–12h IV/IM
>7 days, <1.2 kg:	100 mg/kg/24 hr ÷ q12h IV/IM
≥1.2 kg:	150 mg/kg/24 hr ÷ q8h IV/IM
Infant/child (<50 kg):	100–200 mg/kg/24 hr ÷ q6–8h IV/IM
Meningitis:	200 mg/kg/24 hr ÷ q6h IV/IM (max. dose: 12 g/24 hr)
Adults (≥50 kg):	1–2 g/dose ÷ q6–8h IV/IM (max. dose: 12 g/24 hr)
IV dilution:	
Direct IV:	max. concentration: 100 mg/mL (200 mg/mL CVL) over 3–5 min
Intermittent infusion:	20–60 mg/mL over 10–30 min
Compatibility:	D_5W, NS, LR

Nursing Implications

Use with caution in children with pencillin sensitivity and in impaired renal function. Can cause neutropenia; thrombocytopenia; eosinophilia; positive Coombs' test; and transient increased blood urea nitrogen (BUN), creatinine, and liver enzymes.

cefoxitin (Mefoxin)

Indications

(antibiotic; second-generation cephalosporin)

Used in treatment of skin, bone, joint, respiratory tract, urinary tract, intraabdominal, and gynecologic infections.

Administration

Infant/child:	80–160 mg/kg/24 hr ÷ q4–8h IV/IM
Adult:	4–12 g/24 hr ÷ q6–8h IV/IM (max. dose: 12 g/24 hr)
IV dilution:	
Direct IV:	max. concentration: 100 mg/mL over 3–5 min
Intermittent infusion:	10–40 mg/mL over 10–60 min
Compatibility:	D_5W, NS, LR, $D_{10}W$

Nursing Implications

Use with caution in children with penicillin sensitivity and in impaired renal function. Can cause HA; fever; rash; pseudomembranous colitis; nausea; vomiting; diarrhea; positive direct Coombs' test; transient elevation of BUN, creatinine, and LFTs; and transient leukopenia, thrombocytopenia, neutropenia, anemia, and eosinophilia.

cefprozil (Cefzil)

Indications

(antibiotic; second-generation cephalosporin)

Used in treatment of respiratory tract and skin infections and OM.

Administration

OM: 6 mo–12 yr:	30 mg/kg/24 hr ÷ q12h PO
Pharyngitis/tonsillitis: 2–12 yr:	15 mg/kg/24 hr ÷ q12h PO
Other: ≥12 yr:	500–100 mg/24 hr ÷ q12–24h PO (max. dose: 1 g/24 hr)

Nursing Implications

Absorption not affected by food. Can cause HA, rash, nausea, vomiting, and serum sickness–like reactions.

ceftazidime (Fortaz, Ceptaz)

Indications

(antibiotic; third-generation cephalosporin)

Same as in cefoxitin, plus septicemia, meningitis, osteomyelitis, and cystic fibrosis (CF).

Administration

Neonate:	
≤7 days:	100 mg/kg/24 hr ÷ q12h IV/IM
>7 days, <1.2 kg:	100 mg/kg/24 hr ÷ q12h IV/IM
≥1.2 kg:	150 mg/kg/24 hr ÷ q8h IV/IM
Infant/child:	90–150 mg/kg/24 hr ÷ q8h IV/IM
Meningitis:	150 mg/kg/24 hr ÷ q8h IV/IM
CF:	150 mg/kg/24 hr ÷ q8h IV/IM
Adult:	2–6 g/24 hr ÷ q8–12h IV/IM (max. dose: 6 g/24 hr)
IV dilution:	
Direct IV:	max. concentration: 100 mg/mL over 3–5 min
Intermittent infusion (preferred):	≤40 mg/mL over 15–30 min
Compatibility:	D_5W, NS, LR

Nursing Implications

See cefoxitin.

ceftriaxone (Rocephin)

Indications

(antibiotic; third-generation cephalosporin)

Used in treatment of sepsis; meningitis; lower respiratory tract infections; skin, bone, and joint infections; documented or suspected gonococcal infections; and resistant OM.

Administration

Neonate:	
Gonococcal ophthalmia or prophylaxis:	25–50 mg/kg/dose × 1 IV/IM (max. dose: 125 mg/dose)
Infant/child:	50–75 mg/kg/24 hr ÷ q12–24h IV/IM
	80–100 mg/kg/24 hr ÷ q12–24h IV/IM recommended for infections outside the CSF caused by penicillin-resistant pneumococci
Meningitis:	100 mg/kg/24 hr ÷ q12h IV/IM (max. dose: 4 g/24 hr)
Acute OM:	50 mg/kg IM × 1 (max. dose: 1 g)
Adult:	1–4 g/24 hr ÷ q12–24h IV/IM (max. dose: 4 g/24 hr)

Gonococcal prophylaxis/
uncomplicated gonorrhea: 125 mg IM × 1 dose
Chancroid: 250 mg IM × 1 dose
IV dilution:
Direct IV: max. concentration: 40 mg/mL over 3–5 min
Intermittent infusion (preferred): 10–40 mg/mL over 10–30 min
Compatibility: D_5W, NS, LR, $D_{10}W$

Nursing Implications

Use with caution in children with penicillin sensitivity or impaired renal function. May cause jaundice, reversible cholelithiasis, HA, nausea, vomiting, and diarrhea.

cefuroxime, cefuroxime axetil (Zinacef IV/IM, Ceftin PO)

Indications

(antibiotic; second-generation cephalosporin)

Used same as other cephalosporins. Not recommended for meningitis. PO form used to treat OM, pharyngitis, tonsillitis, and impetigo.

Administration

Neonate: 20–60 mg/kg/24 hr ÷ q12h IV/IM
Infant/child: 75–100 mg/kg/24 hr ÷ q8h IV/IM (max. dose: 6 g/24 hr)
Pharyngitis:
Suspension: 20 mg/kg/24 hr ÷ q12h PO (max. dose: 500 mg/24 hr)
Tablet: 125 mg q12h
OM/impetigo:
Suspension: 30 mg/kg/24 hr ÷ q12h PO (max. dose: 1 g/24 hr)
Tablet: 250 mg q12h
Adult: 750 mg–1.5 g/dose q8h IV/IM (max. dose: 9 g/24 hr)
250–500 mg b.i.d. PO (max. dose: 1 g/24 hr)
IV dilution:
Direct IV: max. concentration: 100 mg/mL over 3–5 min

Intermittent infusion (preferred):	≤30 mg/mL over 15–30 min
Compatibility:	D_5W, NS, LR, $D_{10}W$

Nursing Implications

Use with caution in children with penicillin sensitivity or impaired renal function. May cause thrombophlebitis at infusion site. Tablets and suspension are not equivalent and cannot be substituted on a mg-to-mg basis. Administer suspension with food. Most common side effects are HA, rash, nausea, vomiting, and diarrhea.

cephalexin (Keflex)

Indications

(antibiotic; first-generation cephalosporin)

Used to treat skin infections including impetigo; group A beta hemolytic streptococcal infections; OM; and infections of the respiratory tract, bone, and GU tract.

Administration

Infant/child:	25–100 mg/kg/24 hr ÷ q6–12h PO
Adult:	1–4 g/24 hr ÷ q6–12h PO (max. dose: 4 g/24 hr)

Nursing Implications

Use with caution in children with penicillin sensitivity and in impaired renal function. Can cause GI disturbance, HA, and rash. Absorbed best on an empty stomach but can be given with food or milk to decrease GI irritation. Less frequent dosing such as q8–12h can be used for uncomplicated infections.

cephalothin (Keflin)

Indications

(antibiotic; first-generation cephalosporin)

Used to treat respiratory tract, skin, urinary tract, bone, and joint infections; endocarditis; and septicemia.

Administration

Neonate:	
≤7 days, <2 kg:	40 mg/kg/24 hr ÷ q12h IV
≥2 kg:	60 mg/kg/24 hr ÷ q8h IV
>7 days, <2 kg:	40–60 mg/kg/24 hr ÷ q8–12h IV
≥2 kg:	80 mg/kg/24 hr ÷ q6h IV

Infant/child:	80–160 mg/kg/24 hr ÷ q4–6h IV or deep IM
Adult:	2–12 g/24 hr ÷ q4–6h IV/IM (max. dose: 12 g/24 hr)
IV dilution:	
Direct IV:	max. concentration: 100 mg/mL over 3–5 min
Intermittent infusion:	≤100 mg/mL over 30–60 min
Compatibility:	D_5W, NS, LR, SW

Nursing Implications

Can cause HA, rash, nausea, vomiting, diarrhea, and severe phlebitis, especially with doses >6 g/24 hr for >3 days.

cetirizine (Zyrtec)

Indications

(antihistamine, less sedating)

Used in perennial and seasonal allergic rhinitis and in chronic idiopathic urticaria.

Administration

Child 2–5 yr:	Initial dose 2.5 mg q.d. PO, if needed can increase dose to max. dose of 5 mg/24 hr PO
≥6 yr–adult:	5–10 mg q.d. PO

Nursing Implications

May cause HA, pharyngitis, GI symptoms, dry mouth, and sedation. Give dose at bedtime if sedation is a problem.

chloral hydrate (Noctec)

Indications

(sedative; hypnotic)

Used for short-term sedation and before procedures.

Administration

Child:	
Sedative:	25–50 mg/kg/24 hr q6–8h PO/PR (max. dose: 500 mg)
Procedure:	25–100 mg/kg/dose PO/PR (max. dose: infant—1 g; child—2 g)
Adult:	
Sedative:	250 mg/dose t.i.d. PO/PR
Hypnotic:	500–1,000 mg/dose PO/PR (max. dose: 2 g/24 hr)

Nursing Implications

Irritating to mucous membranes. Can cause GI irritation, paradoxic excitement, hypotension, and heart and respiratory depression. Can accumulate with repeated use. Do not use in children with liver or renal impairment. Use with caution in children with heart disease or those on furosemide (IV) or anticoagulants. Peak effects in 30–60 min. Do not exceed 2 wk of chronic use. Sudden withdrawal can cause delirium tremens.

chloramphenicol (Chloromycetin)

Indications

(antibiotic)

Used in treatment of serious skin and soft tissue, intraabdominal, and CNS infections and bacteremia when organisms are resistant to other less toxic antibiotics. Also used in treatment of rickettsial infections such as Rocky Mountain spotted fever and typhus. Topical and ophthalmic routes are used for local management of superficial infections.

Administration

Ophthalmic:	1–2 gtt. or ribbon of ointment in each eye q3–6h
Topical:	Apply to affected area t.i.d.–q.i.d.
Neonate:	
Loading dose:	20 mg/kg IV
Maintenance dose:	
≤7 days:	25 mg/kg/24 hr q.d. IV
>7 days, ≤2 kg:	25 mg/kg/24 hr q.d. IV
>2 kg:	50 mg/kg/24 hr ÷ q12h IV

First maintenance dose should be given 12 hr after loading dose.

Infant/child/adult:	50–75 mg/kg/24 hr IV/PO ÷ q6h
Meningitis:	75–100 mg/kg/24 hr ÷ q6h IV (max. dose: 4 g/24 hr)
IV dilution:	
Direct IV:	max. concentration: 100 mg/mL over 5 min
Intermittent infusion:	≤20 mg/mL over 15–30 min
Compatibility:	D_5W, NS, LR

Nursing Implications

Monitor blood levels. Therapeutic levels: 15–25 mg/L for meningitis; 10–20 mg/L for other infections. PO doses achieve higher levels than IV doses. Use with caution in G6PD deficiency, in renal or hepatic dysfunction, and in neonates. Can cause three major toxicities: bone marrow suppression; gray syndrome of the newborn, characterized by circulatory collapse, hypothermia, coma, and death; and aplastic anemia 3 wk to 12 mo after initial exposure to chloramphenicol. Also can cause HA, rash, diarrhea, vomiting, and anaphylaxis. Because of the major toxicities after both short- and long-term use, chloramphenicol is not used when less toxic agents are effective.

cimetidine (Tagamet)

Indications

(histamine-2 antagonist)

Used for short-term treatment and long-term prophylaxis of duodenal ulcers; treatment of benign gastric ulcers; management of GE reflux; and to inhibit gastric acid secretion.

Administration

Neonate:	5–20 mg/kg/24 hr ÷ q6–12h PO/IV/IM
Infant:	10–20 mg/kg/24 hr ÷ q6h PO/IV/IM
Child:	20–40 mg/kg/24 hr ÷ q6h PO/IV/IM
Adult:	300 mg/dose q.i.d., 400 mg/dose b.i.d., *or* 800 mg/dose q.h.s. PO/IV/IM
Ulcer prophylaxis:	400–800 mg q.h.s. PO (max. dose: 2,400 mg/24 hr)
IV dilution:	
Direct IV:	max. concentration: 15 mg/mL over 15 min
Intermittent infusion (preferred):	6 mg/mL over 15–30 min
Compatibility:	D_5W, NS, LR, $D_{10}W$

Nursing Implications

Rapid IV administration can cause hypotension, arrhythmias, cardiac arrest. Also can cause rash, mild diarrhea, nausea and vomiting, myalgia, neutropenia, gynecomastia, elevated LFTs, and dizziness. Do not give PO with antacids.

ciprofloxacin (Cipro, Ciloxan ophthalmic, Cipro HC otic)

Indications

(antibiotic; quinolone)

Used in treatment of documented or suspected pseudomonal or serious drug-resistant infections of the respiratory or urinary tract, skin, bone, joint, eye, and ear.

Administration

Child: 20–30 mg/kg/24 hr ÷ q12h PO (max. dose: 1.5 g/24 hr)
10–20 mg/kg/24 hr ÷ q12h IV (max. dose: 800 mg/24 hr)
CF: 40 mg/kg/24 hr ÷ q12h PO (max. dose: 2 g/24 hr)
30 mg/kg/24 hr ÷ q8h IV (max. dose: 1.2 g/24 hr)
Adult: 250–750 mg/dose q12h PO
200–400 mg/dose q12h IV
Ophthalmic: 1–2 gtt. q2h while awake × 2 days, then 1–2 gtt. q4h while awake × 5 days
Otic (>1 yr)/adult: 3 gtt. to affected ear b.i.d. × 7 days
IV dilution: Not to exceed max. concentration: 2 mg/mL over 60 min
Compatibility: D_5W, NS

Nursing Implications

Can cause GI upset, renal failure. GI symptoms, HA, restlessness, and rash are most common side effects. Use with caution in children <18 years. Can increase effect or toxicity of theophylline, warfarin, and cyclosporin. Do not administer antacids with or within 2–4 hr after PO ciprofloxacin dose. Shake suspension vigorously before administration. IV administration given too quickly can cause swelling, pain, burning, and phlebitis.

clarithromycin (Biaxin)

Indications

(antibiotic; macrolide)

Used in treatment of upper and lower respiratory tract infections, acute OM, and infections of the skin and skin structures, as well as for prophylaxis and treatment of *Mycobacterium avium* complex (MAC) disease in patients with advanced HIV infection, treatment of *Helicobacter pylori* infection, and prophylaxis of bacterial endocarditis in patients who are allergic to penicillin.

Administration

Child:
OM, pharyngitis, pneumonia, sinusitis, skin infection: 15 mg/kg/24 hr ÷ q12h PO
MAC prophylaxis: 15 mg/kg/24 hr ÷ q12h PO
Bacterial endocarditis prophylaxis: 15 mg/kg 1 hr before procedure (max. dose: 1 g/24 hr)
Adult: 250–500 mg/dose q12h PO
MAC prophylaxis: 500 mg/dose q12h PO
Bacterial endocarditis prophylaxis: 500 mg 1 hr before procedure

Nursing Implications

Contraindicated in patients allergic to erythromycin. May cause diarrhea, nausea, abnormal taste, dyspepsia, abdominal discomfort, and HA. May increase carbamazepine, theophylline, and cyclosporin levels. May be administered with food.

clindamycin (Cleocin)

Indications

(antibiotic)

Used in treatment of skin, respiratory tract, intraabdominal, and gynecologic infections; septicemia; and osteomyelitis. Topical used in treatment of severe acne.

Administration

Neonate:	
≤7 days, ≤2 kg:	5 mg/kg/dose ÷ q12h IV/IM
>2 kg:	5 mg/kg/dose ÷ q8h IV/IM
>7 days, <1.2 kg:	5 mg/kg/dose ÷ q12h IV/IM
1.2–2 kg:	5 mg/kg/dose ÷ q8h IV/IM
>2 kg:	5 mg/kg/dose ÷ q6h IV/IM
Child:	10–30 mg/kg/24 hr ÷ q6–8h PO
	25–40 mg/kg/24 hr ÷ q6–8h IV/IM
Adult:	150–450 mg/dose q6–8h PO (max. dose: 1.8 g/24 hr)
	1,200–1,800 mg/24 hr ÷ q6–12h IV/IM (max. dose: 4.8 g/24 hr)
Topical:	Apply to affected area b.i.d.
IV dilution:	max. concentration: 18 mg/mL over 10–60 min
	Do not exceed 30 mg/min
Compatibility:	D_5W, NS, LR

Nursing Implications

Contraindicated in liver impairment and diarrhea. Can cause diarrhea, rash. Rapid infusion can cause cardiac arrest. Not indicated in meningitis. Pseudomembranous colitis may occur up to several weeks after stopping drug. Can also cause Stevens-Johnson syndrome, granulocytopenia, thrombocytopenia, or sterile abscess at injection site.

clonidine (Catapres)

Indications

(antihypertensive; central α-adrenergic agonist)

Used in management of hypertension and as alternate agent for treatment of attention deficit hyperactivity disorder (ADHD).

Administration

Child: 5–7 μg/kg/24 hr ÷ q6–12h PO; increase to 5–25 μg/kg/24 hr at 5- to 7-day intervals as needed (max. dose: 0.9 mg/24 hr)

Adult: 0.1 mg b.i.d. PO initially; increase in 0.1-mg/24 hr increments at weekly intervals until desired response is achieved (max. dose: 2.4 mg/24 hr)

Nursing Implications

OK to give with food. Side effects include dry mouth, dizziness, drowsiness, fatigue, constipation, anorexia, arrhythmias, and hypotension. Must be tapered gradually over 1 wk to discontinue.

clotrimazole (Lotrimin, Mycelex)

Indications

(antifungal)

Used to treat fungal infections of the mouth, skin, and vulvovaginal area.

Administration

Topical:	Apply to skin b.i.d. × 4–8 wk
Vaginal candidiasis (vaginal tabs):	100 mg/dose q.h.s. × 7 days
	200 mg/dose q.h.s. × 3 days *or*
	500 mg/dose × 1 *or*
	1 applicator dose (5 g) of 1% vaginal cream q.h.s. × 7–10 days
>3 yr–adult:	
Thrush:	Slowly dissolve one 10-mg troche in mouth 5x/24 hr × 14 days

Nursing Implications

May cause erythema, blistering, or urticaria with topical use. Also can increase liver enzymes and cause nausea and vomiting when given orally.

codeine (Many brands)

Indications

(narcotic; analgesic; antitussive)

Used to treat mild to moderate pain. Used as an antitussive in smaller doses.

Administration

Analgesic:	
Child:	0.5–1 mg/kg/dose q4–6h PO/IM/SC (max. dose: 60 mg/dose)
Adult:	15–60 mg/dose q4–6h PO/IM/SC
Tylenol with Codeine:	Elixir contains acetaminophen 120 mg and codeine 12 mg/5 mL (7% alcohol)
	Tablets with codeine contain 300 mg acetaminophen/tablet
Tylenol #1:	7.5 mg codeine
Tylenol #2:	15 mg codeine
Tylenol #3:	30 mg codeine
Tylenol #4:	60 mg codeine
Antitussive:	All doses p.r.n.; 1–1.5 mg/kg/24 hr ÷ q4–6h; alternatively dose by age as follows:
Child 2–6 yr:	2.5–5 mg/dose q4–6h PO (max. dose: 30 mg/24 hr)
Child 6–12 yr:	5–10 mg/dose q4–6h PO (max. dose: 60 mg/24 hr)
Adult:	10–20 mg/dose q4–6h PO (max. dose: 120 mg/24 hr)

Nursing Implications

Observe for excessive sedation and respiratory depression. Can also cause nausea, constipation, cramping, hypotension, and pruritus. For best pain-relief effects, use with acetaminophen. Do not use as an antitussive in children <2 yr. Give with food to decrease nausea and GI upset. Can be habit forming. *Do not give IV.*

cotrimoxazole (Bactrim, Septra, Cotrim)

Indications

(antibiotic; sulfonamide derivative)

Used in treatment of bronchitis, shigellosis, typhoid fever, OM, and diarrhea. Used for prophylaxis and treatment of *Pneumocystis carinii* pneumonia (PCP) and UTIs.

Administration

Doses based on trimethoprim (TMP) component:

Minor infections:	
Child:	8–10 mg/kg/24 hr ÷ b.i.d. IV/PO
Adult (>40 kg):	160 mg/dose b.i.d.
UTI prophylaxis:	2–4 mg/kg/24 hr q.d.

Severe infections and PCP:	20 mg/kg/24 hr ÷ q6–8h IV/PO
PCP prophylaxis:	5–10 mg/kg/24 hr ÷ b.i.d. 3 consecutive days/wk (max. dose: 320 mg/24 hr)
IV dilution:	1:25 (5 mL of drug to 125 mL of IV fluid) over 60–90 min *Do not give direct IV*
Compatibility:	D_5W, LR

Nursing Implications

Use cautiously with impaired renal or liver function. Not recommended in infants <2 mo. May cause blood dyscrasias, crystalluria, glossitis, renal or hepatic injury, GI irritation, rash, and Stevens-Johnson syndrome. Can cause hemolysis in patients with G6PD.

cromolyn (Intal, Nasalcrom, Gastrocrom, Crolom)

Indications

(antiallergic agent)

Used as oral inhalation or nebulization prophylactic agent for long-term control of persistent asthma and prevention of allergen- or exercise-induced bronchospasm. Used intranasally to manage seasonal or perennial allergic rhinitis. Ophthalmic used to treat vernal conjunctivitis. Oral route used to treat systemic mastocytosis, food allergy, and inflammatory bowel disease (IBD).

Administration

Spin inhalant:	20 mg q6–8h
Nebulization:	20 mg q6–8h
Nasal:	1 spray each nostril t.i.d.–q.i.d.
MDI:	
Child:	1–2 puffs t.i.d.–q.i.d.
Adult:	2–4 puffs t.i.d.–q.i.d.
Ophthalmic:	1–2 gtt. 4–6x/24 hr
Food allergy/IBD:	
Child >2 yr:	100 mg q.i.d. PO; give 15–20 min a.c. and q.h.s. (max. dose: 40 mg/kg/24 hr)
Adult:	200–400 mg q.i.d. PO; give 15–20 min a.c. and q.h.s.
Systemic mastocytosis:	
<2 yr:	20 mg/kg/24 hr ÷ q.i.d. PO (max. dose: 30 mg/kg/24 hr)
2–12 yr:	100 mg q.i.d. PO (max. dose: 40 mg/kg/24 hr)
Adult:	200 mg q.i.d. PO

Nursing Implications

Can cause rash, bronchospasm, cough, and nasal congestion. Oral use can cause HA and diarrhea. Therapeutic response occurs within 2 wk, but may take 4–6 wk to determine maximum benefit. For exercise-induced bronchospasm, give not longer than 1 hr before exercise. Nebulizer solution can be mixed with albuterol.

cyproheptadine (Periactin)

Indications

(antihistamine)

Used in treatment of perennial and seasonal allergic rhinitis and other allergic symptoms including urticaria. Also used as appetite stimulant in anorexia nervosa and as prophylactic for migraines.

Administration

Child:	0.25–0.5 mg/kg/24 hr ÷ q8–12h PO
Adult:	start with 12 mg/24 hr ÷ t.i.d. PO; dosage range 12–32 mg/24 hr ÷ t.i.d. PO
Migraine prophylaxis:	
Child >6 yr:	0.125 mg/kg b.i.d.–t.i.d. PO
6–14 yr:	4 mg b.i.d.–t.i.d.
2–6 yr:	12 mg/24 hr
7–14 yr:	16 mg/24 hr
Adult:	0.5 mg/kg/24 hr

Nursing Implications

Can cause tachycardia, sedation, HA, rash, nausea, and hemolytic anemia. Contraindicated in neonates, in patients on MAO inhibitors, in acute asthma, and in patients with glaucoma or GI/GU obstruction.

deferoxamine mesylate (Desferal)

Indications

(chelating agent)

Used to treat acute iron poisoning and chronic iron overload in children receiving chronic blood transfusions.

Administration

Acute iron poisoning:	
Child:	15 mg/kg/hr IV
	50 mg/kg/dose q6h IM (max. dose: 6 g/24 hr)

Adult:	15 mg/kg/hr IV 1 g × 1, then 0.5 g q4–12h IM (max. dose: 6 g/24 hr)
Chronic iron overload:	
Child:	15 mg/kg/hr IV 20–40 mg/kg/dose q.d. as infusion over 8–12 hr SC
Adult:	0.5–1 g/dose q.d. IM 1–2 g/dose as infusion over 8–24 hr SC
IV dilution:	max. concentration: 250 mg/mL max. rate: 15 mg/kg/hr
Compatibility:	D_5W, NS, LR

Nursing Implications

Contraindicated in anuria. May cause flushing, erythema, urticaria, hypotension, tachycardia, diarrhea, leg cramps, fever, cataracts, and hearing loss. SC not recommended for acute iron poisoning. May cause urine to turn reddish color. Rotate SC sites. Painful lumps with SC administration may indicate rate too fast or needle too close to skin.

desmopressin acetate (DDAVP) (DDAVP, Stimate)

Indications

(vasopressin analog, synthetic; hemostatic agent)

Used in treatment of diabetes insipidus, to control bleeding in certain types of hemophilia, and for primary nocturnal enuresis (bedwetting).

Administration

Diabetes insipidus:	
Child:	0.05 mg b.i.d. PO; titrate to effect
3 mo–12 yr:	5–30 μg/24 hr ÷ q.d.–b.i.d. intranasally
Adult:	0.05 mg b.i.d. PO; titrate to effect, range 0.1–0.2 mg/24 hr ÷ b.i.d.–t.i.d. 10–40 μg/24 hr ÷ q.d.–t.i.d. intranasally; titrate to achieve control of thirst and urination (max. intranasal dose: 40 μg/24 hr)
IV/SC:	2–4 μg/24 hr ÷ b.i.d.
Hemophilia A and von Willebrand's disease:	
Intranasal:	2–4 μg/kg/dose (give 2 hr before procedure)
IV:	0.2–0.4 μg/kg/dose over 15–30 min (give 30 min before procedure)

Nocturnal enuresis (>6 yr):	
PO:	0.2 mg h.s.; titrated to 0.6 mg to achieve desired effect
Intranasal:	20 μg h.s.; range 10–40 μg; divide dose by 2 and put each half dose per nostril
IV dilution:	0.5 μg/mL over 15–30 min
Compatibility:	NS only

Nursing Implications

May cause HA, nausea, hyponatremia, nasal congestion, abdominal cramps, and hypertension. Stimate spray pump must be primed before first use; discard after 25 doses; further doses may be subpotent. Avoid using spray in children <6 yr because of difficulty in titrating dosage.

dexamethasone (Decadron and others)

Implications

(corticosteroid)

Used to manage allergic, inflammatory, hematologic, neoplastic, and autoimmune disorders. Also used in management of cerebral edema and septic shock, as well as before or with first dose of antibiotic in meningitis.

Administration

Cerebral edema:	
Loading dose:	1–2 mg/kg/dose PO/IV/IM × 1
Maintenance:	1–1.5 mg/kg/24 hr ÷ q4–6h PO/IV/IM (max. dose: 16 mg/24 hr)
Airway edema:	0.5–2 mg/kg/24 hr ÷ q6h PO/IV/IM
Croup:	0.6 mg/kg/dose × 1 IV/IM
Antiemetic (chemotherapy induced):	
Initial:	10 mg/m²/dose IV (max.dose: 20 mg)
Subsequent:	5 mg/m²/dose ÷ q6h IV
Anti-inflammatory:	
Child:	0.08–0.3 mg/kg/24 hr ÷ q6–12h PO/IV/IM
Adult:	0.75–9 mg/24 hr ÷ q6–12h PO/IV/IM
Meningitis (>6 wk):	0.6 mg/kg/24 hr ÷ q6h IV × 2 days
IV dilution:	
Direct IV:	4 mg/mL over 1–4 min for doses <10 mg
Intermittent IV:	1 mg/mL over 15–30 min
Compatibility:	D_5W, NS, LR

Nursing Implications

Can cause hypertension, HA, pseudotumor cerebri, adrenal suppression, nausea, vomiting, Cushing's syndrome, muscle weakness, and osteoporosis. May give with food to decrease GI symptoms.

dextroamphetamine (Biphetamine, Dexedrine, Ferdex, Oxydess II)

Indications

(CNS stimulant)

Used to treat ADHD and narcolepsy and for obesity control (in children >12 yr).

Administration

ADHD:

3–5 yr:	2.5 mg/24 hr q AM PO; increase by 2.5 mg/24 hr at weekly intervals (max. dose: 40 mg/24 hr)
≥6 yr:	5 mg/24 hr
Obesity (>12 yr):	5–30 mg/24 hr PO in divided doses of 10–15 mg taken 30–60 min before meals *or* 10- to 15-mg extended-release capsule q AM

Narcolepsy:

6–12 yr:	5 mg/24 hr PO initially; may increase at 5-mg increments qwk until side effects appear (max. dose: 60 mg/day)
>12 yr–adult:	10 mg/24 hr PO initially; may increase at 10-mg increments qwk until side effects appear (max. dose: 60 mg/day)

Nursing Implications

Classified as schedule-II drug under Federal Controlled Substances Act. Monitor pulse and BP. For children with ADHD, obtain caregiver and teacher report about behavioral performance. Many side effects, including insomnia, HA, vomiting, abdominal cramps, restlessness, anorexia, psychosis, dry mouth, and growth failure.

diazepam (Valium and others)

Indications

(anticonvulsant; anxiolytic, benzodiazepine)

Used in management of general anxiety disorders, for sedation, to treat status epilepticus, and as a muscle relaxant.

Administration

Sedative/muscle relaxant:

Child:	0.04–0.2 mg/kg/dose q2–4h IV/IM (max. dose: 0.6 mg/kg in 8 hr)
	0.12–0.8 mg/kg/24 hr ÷ q6–8h PO
Adult:	2–10 mg/dose q3–4h p.r.n. IV/IM
	2–20 mg/dose q6–12h p.r.n. PO

Status epilepticus:

Neonate:	0.3–0.75 mg/kg/dose q15–30 min IV × 2–3 doses
>1 mo:	0.2–0.5 mg/kg/dose q15–30 min IV (max. total dose: <5 yr: 5 mg; ≥5 yr: 10 mg)
IV dilution:	Give undiluted push over 3 min (max. dose: 2 mg/min)

Compatibility: Do not mix with any IV fluids; administer as close to site as possible because it interacts with the plastic IV tubing.

Nursing Implications

Hypotension and respiratory depression can occur. CNS depressants, cimetidine, erythromycin, and valproic acid may enhance effects of diazepam.

dicloxacillin (Dynapen, Pathocil, and others)

Indications

(antibiotic; penicillin, penicillinase-resistant)

Used in treatment of skin and soft tissue infections and pneumonia and as follow-up therapy for osteomyelitis.

Administration

Child (<40 kg):

Mild to moderate infections:	12.5–25 mg/kg/24 hr ÷ q6h PO
Severe infections:	50–100 mg/kg/24 hr ÷ q6h PO
Adult (≥40 kg):	125–500 mg/dose q6h PO (max. dose: 4 g/24 hr)

Nursing Implications

Administer 1–2 hr before or 2 hr after meals. Can cause nausea, vomiting, and diarrhea.

digoxin (Lanoxin)

Implications

(anitarrhythmic agent; inotrope)

Used in treatment of CHF to slow HR in atrial fibrillation and flutter and to end paroxysmal atrial tachycardia. Increases force of myocardial contraction; decreases conduction through sinoatrial (SA) and atrioventricular (AV) nodes. Increases cardiac output.

Administration

Maintenance doses:

Neonate (full term):	8–10 μg/kg/24 hr b.i.d. PO
	6–8 μg/kg/24 hr b.i.d. IV/IM
Child <2 yr:	10–12 μg/kg/24 hr b.i.d. PO
	7.5–9 μg/kg/24 hr b.i.d. IV/IM
2–10 yr:	8–10 μg/kg/24 hr b.i.d. PO
	6–8 μg/kg/24 hr b.i.d. IV/IM
>10 yr (<100 kg):	2.5–5 μg/kg/24 hr q.d. PO
	2–3 μg/kg/24 hr q.d. IV/IM
IV dilution:	Undiluted or diluted at least 4-fold slowly over 5–10 min
	max. concentration: Child: 100 μg/mL; adult: 250 μg/mL
Compatibility:	D_5W, NS, $D_{10}W$

Nursing Implications

Children started on digoxin are given total digitalizing dose (TDD), which is approximately 4 × maintenance dose initially, as follows: 1/2 the TDD, then 1/4 the TDD q8–18h × 2, then ECG is obtained to assess for toxicity. If tolerated, client is started on maintenance dose as listed previously. Check apical pulse for 1 full min before administration. Hold dose and check with doctor if HR <90–100 bpm for an infant, 70 bpm for a child, and 60 bpm for an adult, or according to hospital policy. IV dose should be double checked before administering. Less than 4-fold dilution can cause precipitation. Therapeutic levels: 0.8–2.0 ng/mL. Most common side effects in infants and children are nausea and vomiting. IM route usually not recommended because of local irritation, pain, and tissue damage.

diphenhydramine (Benadryl)

Indications

(antihistamine)

Used in treatment of allergic symptoms caused by histamine release such as nasal allergies and allergic dermatosis, for mild nighttime sedation, for motion-sickness prevention, and as an antitussive. Also used in anaphylaxis and phenothiazine overdose (OD).

Administration

Child:	5 mg/kg/24 hr ÷ q6h PO/IV/IM (max. dose: 300 mg/24 hr)
Adult:	10–50 mg/dose q4–8h PO/IV/IM (max. dose: 400 mg/24 hr)
Anaphylaxis/phenothiazine OD:	1–2 mg/kg IV
IV dilution:	max. concentration: 25 mg/mL over 10–15 min max. rate: 25 mg/min
Compatibility:	D_5W, NS, LR

Nursing Implications

Contraindicated in acute asthma. Use cautiously in liver impairment. Can cause drowsiness, dizziness, and dry mouth. May cause paradoxical excitement in children.

divalproex sodium (Depakote)

Indications

(anticonvulsant)

See valproic acid (page 142) for indications, administration, and nursing implications. Preferred over valproic acid for patients on ketogenic diet.

docusate sodium (Colace, Senokot-S, and others)

Indications

(stool softener; laxative)

Used in patients who should avoid straining during defecation; in constipation associated with hard, dry stools; and to soften ear wax.

Administration

<3 yr:	10–40 mg/24 hr ÷ q.d.–q.i.d. PO
3–6 yr:	20–60 mg/24 hr ÷ q.d.–q.i.d. PO
6–12 yr:	40–150 mg/24 hr ÷ q.d.–q.i.d. PO
>12 yr:	50–500 mg/24 hr ÷ q.d.–q.i.d. PO
Rectal (older children/adults):	Add 50–100 mg oral solution to enema fluid
Ear:	Use a few drops of 10-mg/mL solution in ear canal to soften wax

Nursing Implications

Prolonged use leads to dependence. Oral dose may take 1–3 days of therapy to be effective. Oral solution better tolerated with milk or fruit juice.

ELA-*Max* (lidocaine 4%)

Indications

(topical analgesic)

Used as topical anesthetic on normal, intact skin for dermal anesthesia before painful procedures. May also be used for temporary relief of pain associated with minor cuts and abrasions of skin; minor burns, including sunburn; minor skin irritation; and insect bites. Is a 4% lidocaine cream in a liposomal vehicle. Liposomal encapsulation uses lipid bilayers to deliver anesthetic into dermis.

Administration

For topical use only. Thick layer of ELA-*Max* cream is applied to intact skin. Recommended application time is 15–45 min, with no occlusive dressing required.

Maximum areas for application in children:

≤10 kg:	100 cm² (4 × 4 in.)
10–20 kg:	600 cm² (10 × 10 in.)

Nursing Implications

Explain to child that ELA-*Max* is like a "magic cream that takes hurt away."

Cream is contraindicated in areas where drug could migrate into ears or eyes and on nonintact skin.

EMLA (eutectic mixture of lidocaine 2.5% and prilocaine 2.5%)

Indications

(topical analgesic)

Used as topical anesthetic on normal, intact skin for local anesthesia before painful procedures such as IV insertion, lumbar puncture, implanted port access, peripherally inserted central catheter (PICC) line insertion, superficial biopsy, pacing wire removal, bone marrow aspiration, and IM/SC injections. As of March 11, 1999, U.S. Food and Drug Administration (FDA) has approved use of EMLA for infants born at 37 weeks' gestational age. In infants, EMLA has been safely used for newborn circumcision, IM injections of vitamin K and hepatitis B vaccine, and heel lancing for genetic testing or bilirubin levels.

Administration

For topical use only. Apply thick layer of cream to intact skin. Cover with transparent occlusive dressing (such as Tegaderm). Cream should remain as dollop. Leave in place 1 hr for minor procedures (i.e., superficial punctures) and 2 hr for major procedures (i.e., deep penetration). After removing dressing, wipe cream from skin. Test skin sensitivity and reapply if necessary. In addition to EMLA cream, the EMLA Anesthetic Disc is available, which contains 1 g of EMLA emulsion. The peel-and-stick disc is excellent for home use to anesthetize small areas (2–in. diameter).

Maximum areas for application in children:	
<5 kg:	10 cm^2 (1.25 × 1.25 in.)
5–10 kg:	100 cm^2 (4 × 4 in.)
10–20 kg:	600 cm^2 (10 × 10 in.)
>20 kg:	2,000 cm^2 (18 × 18 in.)

Nursing Implications

Explain to child that EMLA is like a "magic cream that takes hurt away." Cream is contraindicated in areas where drug could migrate into eyes or ears, on nonintact skin or mucous membranes, in congenital or idiopathic methemoglobinemia, and in children receiving methemoglobinemia-inducing agents. Methemoglobin is a dysfunctional form of hemoglobin resulting in reduced oxygen-carrying capacity of blood and leading to cyanosis and hypoxemia. No cases of this complication have been reported in children taking acetaminophen and using EMLA. In fact, there is no evidence that acetaminophen is a methemoglobinemia-inducing drug in humans.

erythromycin (Many brands)

Indications

(antibiotic; macrolide)

Used in treatment of upper and lower respiratory tract infections, skin infections, pertussis, diphtheria, rheumatic fever, Lyme disease, and chlamydia. Topical preparation used to treat acne. Ophthalmic used to prevent neonatal gonococcal or chlamydial ophthalmia.

Administration

Neonate:	
<1.2 kg:	20 mg/kg/24 hr ÷ q12h PO
≥1.2 kg, 0–7 days:	20 mg/kg/24 hr ÷ q12h PO
>7 days:	30 mg/kg/24 hr ÷ q8h PO
Chlamydial conjunctivitis and pneumonia:	50 mg/kg/24 hr ÷ q6h PO × 14 days
Child:	30–50 mg/kg/24 hr ÷ q6–8h PO (max. dose: 2 g/24 hr) 20–50 mg/kg/24 hr ÷ q6h IV
Adult:	1–4 g/24 hr ÷ q6h PO (max. dose: 4 g/24 hr) 15–20 mg/kg/24 hr ÷ q6h IV (max. dose: 4 g/24 hr)
Rheumatic fever prophylaxis:	500 mg/24 hr ÷ q12h PO
Pertussis (Use Estolate salt):	50 mg/kg/24 hr ÷ q6h PO × 14 days
Ophthalmic:	Apply 0.5-in. ribbon to affected eye b.i.d.–q.i.d.
IV dilution:	max. concentration: 5 mg/mL Usual: 1–2.5 mg/mL over 20–60 min *Do not give IV push.*
Compatibility:	D_5W, NS

Nursing Implications

Nausea, vomiting, and abdominal cramps common. Give after meals. Use with caution in liver disease. Can increase digoxin, theophylline, carbamazepine, cyclosporin, and methylprednisolone levels. Ventricular arrhythmias, prolongation of Q-T interval, bradycardia, and hypotension associated with IV use. Prolonging IV infusion duration over ≥60 min has been recommended to decrease cardiotoxic effects.

erythromycin ethylsuccinate and sulfisoxazole acetyl (Pediazole)

Indications

(antibiotic; macrolide and sulfonamide derivative)

Used in treatment of bacterial infections of the upper and lower respiratory tract and OM.

Administration

Child: 50 mg/kg/24 hr erythromycin and 150 mg/kg/24 hr of sulfisoxazole ÷ q6h PO *or* 1.25 mL/kg/24 hr ÷ q6h PO (max. dose: 2 g erythromycin and 6 g sulfisoxazole/24 hr)

Nursing Implications

Same as erythromycin. Not recommended in infants <2 mo.

fentanyl (Actiq, Duragesic, Fentanyl Transdermal, Sublimaze)

Indications

(narcotic; analgesic; sedative)

Short-acting analgesic used during anesthesia and in immediate postoperative period. May also be used transdermally to manage chronic pain.

Administration

IV/IM:	1–2 μg/kg/dose q30–60min p.r.n.
Continuous IV:	1 μg/kg/hr; titrate dose to effect; usual range: 1–3 μg/kg/hr
IV:	For conscious sedation, dose is 0.5–1 μg/kg
Transmucosal lozenge:	10–15 μg/kg for preoperative sedation (not to be used in children <15 kg) 20–40 min before procedure
Transdermal patch:	25 μg/hr for children >12 years and 50 kg Apply to upper torso over dry skin (safety and efficacy have not been established in children <12 yr)
IV dilution:	Undiluted slow push over 3–5 min, or if >5 μg/kg over 5–10 min Also can give by continuous infusion

Nursing Implications

Classified as schedule-II drug under FCS Act. Instruct child to suck (not chew) lozenge for 10–20 min. Drug should be used only in monitored setting equipped for emergency airway and ventilation management. Oxygen saturation monitor should be in place. Child should be kept in bed with side rails up during administration. Can cause respiratory depression, apnea, hypotension, bradycardia, and nausea and vomiting.

folic acid/folate (Folvite and others)

Indications

(water-soluble vitamin)

Used to stimulate production of red blood cells, white blood cells, and platelets in anemias caused by folate deficiency. Also reduces risk of neural tube deficits in infants if mother takes before and during pregnancy.

Administration

Folic acid deficiency:

PO/IV/IM/SC	Initial Dose	Maintenance
<1 yr:	15 μg/kg/dose; (max. dose: 50 μg/24 hr)	30–45 μg/24 hr
1–10 yr:	1 mg/dose	0.1–0.4 mg/24 hr q.d.
11 yr–adult:	1–3 mg/dose ÷ q.d.–t.i.d.	0.5 mg/24 hr q.d.
Pregnant/lactating:		0.8 mg/24 hr q.d.
IV dilution:	0.1 mg/mL	

Compatibility: D_5W, NS, SW

Nursing Implications

Urine may appear more yellow. If given IM, give deep IM. Can cause rash, slight flushing, irritability, and GI upset. Normal levels: serum >3 ng/mL.

furosemide (Lasix, Furomide MD, and others)

Indications

(loop diuretic)

Used in management of edema from CHF or hepatic or renal disease and in treatment of hypertension.

Administration

Neonate:	0.5–1 mg/kg/dose q8–24 hr PO/IV/IM (max. dose: 6 mg/kg/dose PO; 2 mg/kg/dose IV)
Infant/child:	0.5–2 mg/kg/dose q6–12 hr PO/IV/IM (max. dose: 6 mg/kg/dose)
Adult:	20–80 mg/24 hr ÷ q6–12h (max. dose: 600 mg/24 hr)
Continuous IV infusion:	
Child/adult:	0.05 mg/kg/hr; titrate to effect
IV dilution:	Undiluted over 1–2 min (max. dose: 0.5 mg/kg/min (<120 mg) *or* 4 mg/min (>120 mg)

	Intermittent infusion 1–2 mg/mL (max. dose: 10 mg/mL) over 10–15 min
Compatibility:	D_5W, NS, LR

Nursing Implications

Use cautiously in liver disease. May cause hypokalemia. Observe for dehydration. Oral solutions can cause diarrhea.

gentamicin (Garamycin)

Indications

(antibiotic; aminoglycoside)

Used in treatment of serious gram-negative bacterial infections of the respiratory tract, skin, bone, abdomen, urinary tract, and CNS; endocarditis; and septicemia.

Administration

Neonate:	Doses based on gestational age, postnatal age, and weight. Consult pharmacy and/or pediatric drug reference.
Child:	6–7.5 mg/kg/24 hr ÷ q8h IV/IM
Adult:	3–6 mg/kg/24 hr ÷ q8h IV/IM
CF:	7.5–10.5 mg/kg/24 hr ÷ q8h IV/IM
IV dilution:	1–2 mg/mL
	max. concentration: 10 mg/mL over 30–60 min
	Can give by direct injection over 15 min, not to exceed 10 mg/mL
Compatibility:	D_5W, NS, LR

Nursing Implications

Ototoxic and nephrotoxic. Monitor levels. Therapeutic levels: peak: 6–10 mg/L (8–10 in pulmonary infections); trough: <2 mg/L. Administer other IV antibiotics at least 1 hr before or after gentamicin.

glucagon (Glucagon)

Indications

(antihypoglycemic agent)

Used in management of hypoglycemia.

Administration

Neonate/infant:	0.025–0.3 mg/kg/dose q30min p.r.n. IV/IM/SC (max. dose: 1 mg/dose)

Child:	0.03–0.1 mg/kg/dose q20min p.r.n. IV/IM/SC (max. dose: 1 mg/dose)
Adult:	0.5–1 mg/dose q20min p.r.n. IV/IM/SC
IV dilution:	
Direct IV:	Dilute with manufacturer's diluent, resulting in 1-mg/mL concentration. If doses >2 mg are used, dilute with SW instead of diluent.
Compatibility:	All dextrose solutions; will precipitate with NS

Nursing Implications

High doses have cardiac stimulatory effect and have been used in β-blocker overdoses. Can cause nausea, vomiting, urticaria, and respiratory distress.

griseofulvin (Grifulvin V, Grisactin, Fulvicin, Gris-PEG)

Indications

(antifungal agent)

Used in treatment of tinea infections of the skin, hair, and nails.

Administration

Microsize:	
Child:	10–20 mg/kg/24 hr ÷ q.d.–b.i.d. PO
Adult:	500–1,000 mg/24 hr ÷ q.d.–b.i.d. PO (max. dose: 1 g/24 hr)
Ultramicrosize:	
Child >2 yr:	5–10 mg/kg/24 hr ÷ q.d.–b.i.d. PO
Adult:	330–750 mg/24 hr ÷ q.d.–b.i.d. PO (max. dose: 750 mg/24 hr)

Nursing Implications

Give with milk, eggs, or fatty foods to increase absorption. Usual treatment period 4–6 wk for tinea capitis, 4–6 mo for tinea unguium. May cause leukopenia. Monitor hematologic, renal, and hepatic function, especially for courses >4–6 wk. May decrease effectiveness of oral contraceptive pills (OCPs).

hydroxyzine (Atarax, Vistaril)

Indications

(antihistamine; anxiolytic)

Used in treatment of anxiety, for preoperative sedation, and as an antiemetic and antipruritic.

Administration

Child: 2 mg/kg/24 hr ÷ q6–8h PO
0.5–1 mg/kg/dose q4–6h p.r.n. IM
Adult: 25–100 mg/dose q4–6h p.r.n. PO/IM (max. dose: 600 mg/24 hr)

Nursing Implications

Potentiates barbiturates, meperidine, and other depressants. Can cause dry mouth, drowsiness, tremor, convulsions, blurred vision, and hypotension. IV not recommended but has been administered by slow IV to oncology patients via CVLs without problems.

ibuprofen (Motrin, Advil, and others)

Indications

(NSAID)

Used in management of inflammatory disorders such as juvenile rheumatoid arthritis (JRA) and as analgesic for mild to moderate pain. Also used for dysmenorrhea, gout, and fever.

Administration

Child:
- Analgesic/antipyretic: 5–10 mg/kg/dose q6–8h PO (max. dose: 40 mg/kg/24 hr PO)
- JRA: 30–50 mg/kg/24 hr ÷ q6h PO (max. dose: 2,400 mg/24 hr PO)

Adult:
- Inflammatory disease: 400–800 mg/dose q6–8h PO
- Pain/fever/dysmenorrhea: 200–400 mg/dose q4–6h PO (max. dose: 3.2 g/24 hr PO)

Nursing Implications

Use with caution in liver and renal impairment. Can cause nausea, vomiting, rash, and ocular problems. Also can cause granulocytopenia and anemia and inhibit platelet aggregation. May increase serum levels and effects of digoxin, methotrexate, and lithium. May decrease effects of antihypertensives, furosemide, and thiazide diuretics. GI problems can be lessened by administering with milk.

imipramine (Tofranil, Janimine)

Indications

(antidepressant, tricyclic)

Used to treat various forms of depression, enuresis in children, and as analgesic for certain chronic and neuropathic pain.

Administration

Antidepressant:

Child:	Initial: 1.5 mg/kg/24 hr ÷ t.i.d. PO; increase 1–1.5 mg/kg/24 hr q3–4days (max. dose: 5 mg/kg/24 hr)
Adolescent:	Initial: 25–50 mg/24 hr ÷ q.d.–t.i.d. PO; doses >100 mg/24 hr usually not needed
Adult:	Initial: 75–100 mg/24 hr ÷ t.i.d. PO/IM (max. dose: 100 mg/24 hr)
	Maintenance: 50–300 mg/24 hr q h.s. PO (max. PO dose: 300 mg/24 hr)
Enuresis (≥6 yr):	Initial: 10–25 mg q h.s.
	Increment: 10–25 mg/dose at 1- to 2-wk intervals until max. dose for age or desired effect achieved. Continue for 2–3 mo, then taper slowly. (max. dose: 6–12 yr: 50 mg/24 hr; 12–14 yr: 75 mg/24 hr)
Chronic pain:	Initial: 0.2–0.4 mg/kg/dose q h.s. PO; increase 50% q2–3days (max. dose: 1–3 mg/kg/dose q h.s. PO)

Nursing Implications

Can cause hypotension, sedation, urinary retention, constipation, dry mouth, dizziness, drowsiness, and arrhythmia. PO route preferred. *Do not discontinue abruptly in patients receiving long-term high-dose therapy.*

ipecac (Ipecac syrup)

Indications

(emetic agent)

Used to treat drug OD and certain poisonings by producing emesis.

Administration

Child 6–12 mo:	10 mL per dose followed by 10–20 mL/kg of water
Child 1–5 yr:	15 mL per dose followed by 120 mL of water
Child ≥5 yr–adult:	30 mL per dose followed by 200–300 mL of water

Can be repeated one time if child does not vomit in 30 min.

Ipecac syrup differs from ipecac fluid-extract, which is 14x more potent and can lead to death.

Nursing Implications

Assess what child ingested and time of ingestion. Assess level of consciousness; administer to conscious patients only. Position child upright or on side to prevent aspiration. Vomiting should subside within 3 hr. May cause GI irritation, cardiotoxicity, and myopathy. Not recommended for children

<6 mo. Do not give if child has ingested caustic substances such as lye. Avoid use of milk because it delays action of drug. Carbonated beverages decrease effectiveness of ipecac.

ipratropium bromide (Atrovent)

Indications

(anticholinergic agent)

Bronchodilator used in treatment of bronchospasm associated with asthma, chronic obstructive pulmonary disease (COPD), bronchitis, and emphysema. Also used for symptomatic relief of rhinorrhea associated with allergic and nonallergic rhinitis.

Administration

Inhaler:

<12 yr:	1–2 puffs t.i.d.–q.i.d.
≥12 yr:	2–3 puffs q.i.d. up to 12 puffs/24 hr

Nebulized:

Neonate:	25 μg/kg/dose t.i.d.
Infant/child:	250 μg/dose t.i.d.–q.i.d.
>12 yr–adult:	250–500 μg/dose t.i.d.–q.i.d.

Nasal spray:

>12 yr–adult:	2 sprays per nostril b.i.d.–t.i.d.

Nursing Implications

Use with caution in patients with narrow angle glaucoma and bladder neck obstruction. May cause anxiety, dizziness, HA, GI discomfort, and cough with inhaled and nebulized doses. Nasal spray can cause nasal congestion and dry mouth. Shake inhaler well before use. Use spacer in children <8 yr. Nebulized solution can be mixed with albuterol.

iron (Fe) (Fer-In-Sol and others)

Indications

(oral iron supplements)

Used in prevention and treatment of iron-deficiency anemias.

Administration

Treatment:

Preterm:	2–4 mg elemental Fe/kg/24 hr ÷ q.d.–b.i.d. PO (max. dose: 15 mg elemental Fe/24 hr)
Child:	3–6 mg elemental Fe/kg/24 hr ÷ q.d.–t.i.d. PO
Adult:	60 mg elemental Fe b.i.d.–q.i.d.

Prevention:

Preterm:	2 mg elemental Fe/kg/24 hr
Term/child:	1–2 mg elemental Fe/kg/24 hr (max. dose: 15 mg elemental Fe/24 hr)
Adult:	60–100 mg elemental Fe/24 hr PO ÷ q.d.–b.i.d.

Nursing Implications

Liquid preparations stain teeth. Use dropper or straw to administer. Less GI irritation if given with or after meals. Do not give with milk or milk products. May cause constipation, dark stools, nausea, and epigastric pain.

kanamycin (Kantrex)

Indications

(antibiotic; aminoglycoside)

Used in treatment of gram-negative bacillary and staphylococcal infections of bone, respiratory tract, skin, and abdomen; complicated UTIs; endocarditis; and septicemia.

Administration

Neonate:	
<7 days, <2 kg:	15 mg/kg/24 hr ÷ q12h IV/IM
≥2 kg:	20 mg/kg/24 hr ÷ q12h IV/IM
≥7 days, <2 kg:	22.5 mg/kg/24 hr ÷ q8h IV/IM
≥2 kg:	30 mg/kg/24 hr ÷ q8h IV/IM
Infant/child:	15–30 mg/kg/24 hr ÷ q8–12h IV/IM
Adult:	15 mg/kg/24 hr ÷ q8–12h IV/IM
PO for GI bacterial overgrowth:	150–250 mg/kg/24 hr ÷ q6h (max. dose: 4 g/24 hr)
IV dilution:	2.5–5 mg/mL over 30–60 min *Do not give IV push.* 37.5 mg/mL via CVL
Compatibility:	D_5W, NS, LR, $D_{10}W$

Nursing Implications

Renal toxicity and ototoxicity may occur. Poorly absorbed orally, so only used PO to treat GI bacterial overgrowth. Therapeutic levels: peak: 15–30 mg/L; trough: <5–10 mg/L.

ketoconazole (Nizoral)

Indications

(antifungal agent)

Used to treat topical and systemic fungal infections and as suppressive therapy against mucocutaneous candidiasis in HIV patients.

Administration

Oral:

Child ≥2 yr:	3.3–6.6 mg/kg/24 hr q.d.
Adult:	200–400 mg/24 hr q.d. (max. dose: 800 mg/24 hr ÷ b.i.d.)

Topical:	1–2 applications/24 hr
Shampoo:	Twice weekly × 4 wk with at least 3 days between applications, and intermittently as needed to maintain control

Suppressive treatment:

Child:	5–10 mg/kg/24 hr ÷ q.d.–b.i.d. PO
Adolescent/adult:	200 mg/dose q.d. PO

Nursing Implications

Monitor LFTs in long-term use. May cause nausea, vomiting, rash, HA, pruritus and fever. Contraindicated in patients on terfenadine because of possible cardiac arrhythmias. May increase effects and levels of phenytoin, digoxin, cyclosporin, protease inhibitors, and warfarin. Phenobarbital, rifampin, INH, H_2-blockers, antacids, and omeprazole can decrease levels of ketoconazole.

lorazepam (Ativan)

Indications

(benzodiazepine anticonvulsant)

Used in management of anxiety and status epilepticus and for preoperative sedation and amnesia. Also used for antiemetic adjunct therapy.

Administration

Status epilepticus:

Neonate/infant/child/adolescent:	0.05–0.1 mg/kg/dose over 2–5 min IV; may repeat 0.05 mg × 1 in 10–15 min (max. dose: 4 mg/dose)
Adult:	4 mg/dose slowly over 2–5 min IV; may repeat in 5–15 min (total max. dose in 12-hr period is 8 mg)

Antiemetic adjunct:

Child:	0.04–0.08 mg/kg/dose q6h p.r.n. IV (max. single dose: 4 mg)

Anxiolytic/sedation:
- Child: 0.05 mg/kg/dose q4–8h IV/PO *or* IM for procedural sedation (max. dose: 2 mg/dose)
- Adult: 1–10 mg/24 hr ÷ b.i.d.–t.i.d. PO

IV dilution: Do not exceed 2 mg/min or 0.05 mg/kg over 2–5 min

Compatibility: D_5W, NS, SW

Nursing Implications

Injectable form contains 2% benzyl alcohol, which may be toxic to neonates in high doses. Aspirate repeatedly when giving IV to make sure injection is not intraarterial and that perivascular extravasation has not occurred. Injectable form may also be given rectally. May cause respiratory depression, sedation, dizziness, mild ataxia, mood changes, rash, and GI symptoms.

mannitol (Osmitrol, Resectisol)

Indications

(osmotic diuretic)

Used to reduce increased intracranial pressure (ICP) associated with cerebral edema, to promote diuresis in prevention and/or treatment of oliguria or anuria resulting from acute renal failure, to reduce increased ocular pressure, and to promote urinary excretion of toxic substances.

Administration

Anuria/oliguria:
- Test dose (to assess renal function): 0.2 g/kg/dose IV (max. dose: 12.5 g over 3–5 min) If no diuresis, mannitol is discontinued.
- Initial: 0.5–1 g/kg/dose IV
- Maintenance: 0.25–0.5 g/kg/dose q4–6h IV

Cerebral edema: 0.25 g/kg/dose IV over 20–30 min; gradually increased to 1 g/kg/dose if needed

IV administration: In-line filter set (≤5 micron) should always be used for infusion with concentrations ≥20%; test dose given IV push over 3–5 min; for cerebral edema or elevated ICP, administer over 20–30 min

Compatibility: Do not mix with IV fluids. NaCl and KCl can cause precipitation.

Nursing Implications

Do not use solutions that contain crystals. Hot water bath and vigorous shaking may be used to dissolve crystals. Contraindicated in severe renal disease, active intracranial bleed, dehydration, and pulmonary edema. May cause circulatory overload, electrolyte disturbances, hypovolemia, HA, and polydipsia.

meperidine hydrochloride (Demerol and others)

Indications

(narcotic; analgesic)

Used in management of moderate to severe pain. Also used for preoperative sedation.

Administration

PO/IV/IM/SC:	
Child:	1–1.5 mg/kg/dose q3–4h p.r.n. (max. dose: 100 mg)
Adult:	50–150 mg/dose q3–4h p.r.n.
IV dilution:	≤10 mg/mL direct IV slowly over ≥5 min
Intermittent infusion:	1 mg/mL over 15–30 min
Infusion:	0.3–0.7 mg/kg/hr
Compatibility:	D_5W, NS, LR, $D_{10}W$

Nursing Implication

IV dose lower. Contraindicated in patients with cardiac arrhythmias, asthma, and increased ICP. Can cause nausea, vomiting, respiratory depression, smooth muscle spasm, pruritus, palpitations, hypotension, constipation, and lethargy. Continued use decreases effects. Not recommended for chronic use. Dilute PO syrup in water before use.

meropenem (Merrem)

Indications

(antibiotic)

Used in treatment of multidrug-resistant gram-negative and gram-positive aerobic and anaerobic pathogens and for treatment of meningitis; lower respiratory tract, urinary tract, intraabdominal, and skin infections; and sepsis.

Administration

Child ≥3 mo:	60 mg/kg/24 hr ÷ q8h IV
Meningitis:	120 mg/kg/24 hr ÷ q8h IV (max. dose: 6 g/24 hr)
Adult:	
Mild-to-moderate infection:	1.5–3 g/24 hr ÷ q8h IV
Meningitis:	6 g/24 hr ÷ q8h IV
IV dilution:	
Direct IV:	max. concentration: 50 mg/mL over 3–5 min
Intermittent infusion:	50 mg/mL over 15–30 min
Compatibility:	D_5W, NS, SW

Nursing Implications

Probenecid inhibits renal excretion. Safety not established for children <3 mo. Use with caution in patients with history of seizures, with CNS disease or infection, or with decreased renal function. Can cause pseudomembranous colitis; hypotension; rash; nausea and vomiting; diarrhea; neutropenia; increased LFTs, BUN, and creatinine; and dyspnea. Prolonged use may result in superinfection.

methicillin (Staphcillin)

Indications

(antibiotic; penicillin, penicillinase-resistant)

Used in treatment of respiratory tract, skin, bone, joint, and urinary tract infections; and endocarditis, septicemia, and CNS infections caused by susceptible strains of penicillinase-producing *Staphylococcus*.

Administration

Neonate:	
≤7 days, <2 kg:	50–100 mg/kg/24 hr ÷ q12h IV/IM
≥2 kg:	75–150 mg/kg/24 hr ÷ q8h IV/IM
>7 days, <1.2 kg:	50–100 mg/kg/24 hr ÷ q12h IV/IM
1.2–2 kg:	75–150 mg/kg/24 hr ÷ q8h IV/IM
≥2 kg:	100–200 mg/kg/24 hr ÷ q8h IV/IM
Infant >1 mo/child:	150–400 mg/kg/24 hr ÷ q4–6h IV/IM
Adult:	4–12 g/24 hr ÷ q4–6h IV/IM (max. dose: 12 g/24 hr)
IV dilution:	2–20 mg/mL over 15–30 min
Compatibility:	D_5W, NS, LR

Nursing Implications

Administer IM dose deep in large muscle mass using solution with concentration of 500 mg/mL. May cause hematuria, reversible bone marrow depression, hairy tongue, positive Coombs' test and rash, and phlebitis at IV site. Has been associated with interstitial nephritis and hemorrhagic cystitis.

methylphenidate (Ritalin)

Indications

(CNS stimulant)

Used to treat children with ADHD and narcolepsy.

Administration

Initial:	0.3 mg/kg/dose (*or* 2.5–5 mg/dose) given before breakfast and lunch. May increase by 0.1 mg/kg/dose (*or* 5–10 mg/

24 hr) weekly until maintenance dose achieved. May need to give extra afternoon dose.

Maintenance: 0.3–1 mg/kg/24 hr (max. dose: 2 mg/kg/24 hr *or* 60 mg/24 hr)

Nursing Implications

Classified as schedule-II drug under FCS Act. Avoid administration in evening so sleep is not interrupted; however children with severe ADHD may need dose to calm them enough to go to sleep. Assess child's behavior through caregiver and teacher report in regard to concentration ability. Client should be taught to take drug as prescribed. Tapering may be needed when drug is being discontinued. Safe storage is an issue because this drug has potential for street abuse. Should be transported to school by an adult. Child should be observed swallowing pill. High dose may slow growth through appetite suppression. Dose may need to be given after meals for children with appetite suppression. Contraindicated in clients with glaucoma, anxiety disorders, motor tics, and Tourette's syndrome. Can cause insomnia, weight loss, anorexia, rash, nausea, vomiting, abdominal pain, hypertension or hypotension, tachycardia, arrhythmias, palpitations, restlessness, HA, fever, tremor, and thrombocytopenia.

methylprednisolone (Medrol, Solu-Medrol, and others)

Indications

(corticosteroid)

Used in management of chronic inflammatory, allergic, hematologic, neoplastic, and autoimmune diseases.

Administration

Anti-inflammatory/immunosuppressive: 0.5–1.7 mg/kg/24 hr ÷ q6–12h PO/IV/IM

Status asthmaticus:

Child:

Loading: 2 mg/kg/dose IV/IM × 1

Maintenance: 2 mg/kg/24 hr ÷ q6h IV/IM

Adult: 10–250 mg/dose q4–6h IV/IM

IV dilution: Undiluted for push. Max. concentration: 62.5 mg/mL over 3–5 min

Do not administer high dose (15 mg/kg or ≥500 mg/dose) *by IV push.*

Infusion: 2.5–5 mg/mL over 15–60 min

Compatibility: D_5W, NS

Nursing Implications

Monitor BP with IV infusion. Hypotension, cardiac arrhythmia, and sudden death have been reported in patients given high-dose methylprednisolone IV push over <20 min. Do not give acetate form IV. Can cause same type of side effects with long-term use as other corticosteroids. Should never be discontinued abruptly.

metoclopramide (Reglan, Clopra, Maxolon, and others)

Indications

(antiemetic; prokinetic agent)

Used in treatment of GE reflux and in prevention and treatment of nausea and vomiting associated with chemotherapy and postoperatively.

Administration

GE reflux:

Infant/child:	0.1–0.2 mg/kg/dose up to q.i.d. IV/IM/PO (max. dose: 0.8 mg/kg/24 hr)
Adult:	10–15 mg/dose a.c. and q h.s. IV/IM/PO
Antiemetic:	1–2 mg/kg/dose q2–6h IV/IM/PO
IV dilution:	0.2 mg/mL max. concentration: 5 mg/mL over 15–30 min (max. rate 5 mg/min)
Compatibility:	D_5W, NS, LR

Nursing Implications

Contraindicated in GI obstruction, seizure disorder, and pheochromocytoma or in patients receiving drugs likely to cause extrapyramidal symptoms (EPS). May cause EPS, sedation, HA, anxiety, leukopenia, and diarrhea. Give PO dose 30 min a.c. and h.s. for GE reflux.

midazolam (Versed)

Indications

(benzodiazepine)

Used for sedation, anxiolysis, and amnesia before a procedure or anesthesia; conscious sedation for procedures; and continuous sedation of intubated and mechanically ventilated patients. Also sometimes used in status epilepticus.

Administration

Doses titrated to effect under controlled conditions.

Procedural sedation:

PO:

Infant ≥6 mo/child:	single dose, 0.25–0.5 mg/kg/dose; usual dose, 0.5 mg/kg (max. dose: 20 mg)

IM:	
Child:	Usual dose, 0.1–0.15 mg/kg/dose 30–60 min before procedure/surgery (max. total dose: 10 mg)
IV:	
6 mo–5 yr:	0.05–0.1 mg/kg/dose over 2–3 min; may repeat p.r.n. q2–3min (max. total dose: 6 mg)
6–12 yr:	0.025–0.05 mg/kg/dose over 2–3 min; may repeat p.r.n. q2–3min (max. total dose: 10 mg)
>12–16 yr:	Use adult dose up to max. total dose of 10 mg
Adult:	0.5–2 mg/dose over 2 min; may repeat p.r.n. q2–3min (Usual total dose: 2.5–5 mg)
Sedation with mechanical ventilation:	
Intermittent IV:	
Infant/child:	0.05–0.15 mg/kg/dose q1–2h p.r.n.
Continuous IV infusion:	
Neonate:	
<32 wk gestation:	0.5 μg/kg/min
≥32 wk gestation:	1 μg/kg/min
Infant/child:	1–2 μg/kg/min
IV dilution:	1–5 mg/mL over ≥2–5 min *or* by infusion as above
Compatibility:	D_5W or 0.9% NaCl

Nursing Implications

Do not give intraarterially. Give PO on empty stomach. Cardiovascular monitoring recommended. Can cause respiratory depression, hypotension, and bradycardia.

montelukast (Singulair)

Indications

(antiasthmatic; leukotriene receptor antagonist)

Used for prophylaxis and chronic treatment of asthma.

Administration

Child 6–14 yr:	Chew 5-mg chewable tablet q h.s. PO
>15 yr–adult:	10 mg q h.s. PO

Nursing Implications

Contraindicated in phenylketonuric patients. Phenobarbital and rifampin increase clearance of montelukast. Possible side effects include HA, nausea, abdominal pain, diarrhea, dyspepsia, fatigue, dizziness, elevated liver enzymes, cough, laryngitis, pharyngitis, otitis, sinusitis, and viral infections.

morphine sulfate (Many brands)

Indications

(narcotic; analgesic)

Used in management of severe acute and chronic pain. Effective with painful sickle cell crisis and cyanotic spells associated with tetralogy.

Administration

Doses titrated to effect.

Analgesia/tetralogy spells:	
Neonate:	0.05–0.2 mg/kg/dose q4h slow IV/IM/SC
Neonate opiate withdrawal:	0.08–0.2 mg/dose q3–4h slow IV/IM/SC
Infant/child:	0.2–0.5 mg/kg/dose q4–6h p.r.n. PO (immediate release)
	0.3–0.6 mg/kg/dose q12h PO (controlled release)
	0.1–0.2 mg/kg/dose q2–4h p.r.n. IV/IM/SC (max. dose: 15 mg/dose)
Adult:	10–30 mg q4h p.r.n. PO (immediate release)
	15–30 mg q8–12h p.r.n. PO (controlled release)
	2–15 mg/dose q2–6h p.r.n. IV/IM/SC
Continuous IV:	
Neonate:	0.01–0.02 mg/kg/hr
Infant/child:	0.025–2.6 mg/kg/hr
Adult:	0.8–10 mg/hr
IV dilution:	
Direct IV:	0.5–5 mg/mL over 5 min
Intermittent IV:	over 15–30 min
Continuous IV:	0.1–1 mg/mL
Compatibility:	D_5W

Nursing Implications

Give PO dose with food. Rapid IV administration may increase adverse effects. Can cause dependence, CNS and respiratory depression, nausea, vomiting, urinary retention, hypotension, constipation, bradycardia, and increased ICP. Causes histamine release resulting in itching and possible bronchospasm. Assess for sedation and respiratory depression. Naloxone may be used to reverse effects.

nafcillin (Unipen, Nafcil, and others)

Indications

(antibiotic; penicillin, penicillinase resistant)

Used in treatment of penicillinase-producing staphylococci infections of respiratory tract, bone, joints, skin, and urinary tract. Also used in endocarditis, septicemia, and CNS infections.

Administration

Neonate:	
≤7 days, <2 kg:	50 mg/kg/24 hr ÷ q12h IV/IM
≥2 kg:	75 mg/kg/24 hr ÷ q8h IV/IM
>7 days, <1.2 kg:	50 mg/kg/24 hr ÷ q12h IV/IM
1.2–2 kg:	75 mg/kg/24 hr ÷ q8h IV/IM
≥2 kg:	100 mg/kg/24 hr ÷ q6h IV/IM
>7 days:	75 mg/kg/24 hr ÷ q6h IV/IM
Infant/child:	50–100 mg/kg/24 hr ÷ q6h PO
Mild to moderate infections:	50–100 mg/kg/24 hr ÷ q6h IV/IM
Severe infections:	100–200 mg/kg/24 hr ÷ q4–6h IV/IM
Adult:	250–1,000 mg q4–6h PO
	500–2,000 mg q4–6h IV
	500 mg q4–6h IM (max. dose: 12 g/24 hr)
IV dilution:	10–40 mg/mL over 60 min
Compatibility:	D_5W, NS, LR, $D_{10}W$

Nursing Implications

Give PO on empty stomach. Give IM deep into large muscle at 250 mg/mL. High incidence of phlebitis with IV route that can cause tissue sloughing and necrosis. Decrease rate and/or concentration for vein irritation. Sodium bicarbonate may be added to IV dilution to buffer effects. Warm or cold compresses at IV site may help decrease pain during infusion.

naproxen/naproxen sodium (Naprosyn, Anaprox, Aleve [over the counter])

Indications

(NSAID)

Used to manage inflammatory disease and rheumatoid disorders including JRA; acute gout, mild to moderate pain; and dysmenorrhea.

Administration

All doses based on naproxen base.

Child >2 yr:	
Analgesia:	5–7 mg/kg/dose q8–12h PO

JRA: 10–20 mg/kg/24 hr ÷ q12h PO (max. dose: 1,250 mg/24 hr)

Rheumatoid arthritis/ankylosing spondylitis:

Adult: 250–500 mg b.i.d. PO

Dysmenorrhea: 500 mg × 1, then 250 mg q6–8h PO (max. dose: 1,250 mg/24 hr)

Nursing Implications

May cause GI bleeding, thrombocytopenia, heartburn, HA, drowsiness, vertigo, and tinnitus. Use with caution in patients with GI disease, cardiac disease, or renal or hepatic impairment, and in those on anticoagulants. Give with food to decrease GI effects.

nitrofurantoin (Furadantin, Macrodantin)

Indications

(antibiotic)

Used for prevention and treatment of UTIs.

Administration

Child >1 mo:

Treatment: 5–7 mg/kg/24h ÷ q6h PO (max. dose: 400 mg/24 hr)

Prophylaxis: 1–2 mg/kg/dose q h.s. PO (max. dose: 100 mg/24 hr)

Adult:

Treatment: 50–100 mg/dose q6h PO (for dual release: 100 mg/dose q12h PO)

Prophylaxis: 50–100 mg PO q h.s.

Nursing Implications

Can cause nausea, vomiting, HA, and false-positive urine glucose. Contraindicated in severe renal disease and G6PD deficiency, and in infants <1 mo. Give with food or milk.

nystatin (Mycostatin, Nilstat, and others)

Indications

(antifungal agent)

PO, topical, and vaginal treatment of candidal infections.

Administration

Oral:

Preterm infant: 0.5 mL (50,000 U) to each side of mouth q.i.d.

Term infant: 1 mL (100,000 U) to each side of mouth q.i.d.

Child/adult:

Suspension:	4–6 mL (400,000–600,000 U) swish and swallow q.i.d.
Troche:	200,000–400,000 U 4–5x/24 hr
Vaginal:	1 tablet q h.s. × 10 days
Topical:	Apply to affected area b.i.d.–q.i.d.

Nursing Implications

May need to paint on lesions in mouth with cotton swab or clean pacifier with infants. Nipples and pacifiers need to be cleaned thoroughly. Troches must be allowed to dissolve slowly and must not be chewed or swallowed whole. Can cause GI effects. Must continue to treat until 48–72 hr after lesions are gone. For mothers with candidal infection of skin around areola who are breastfeeding their infants, suspension can be rubbed on breasts.

palivizumab (Synagis)

Indications

(monoclonal antibody)

Used to prevent serious disease caused by respiratory syncytial virus (RSV) in infants with chronic lung disease <2 yr old and infants who were born at <35 weeks' gestation and are <12 mo old. Given during RSV season, typically November through April.

Administration

15 mg/kg/dose IM q mo during RSV season

Nursing Implications

IM is only current route. Administer in anterolateral aspect of thigh. Reconstitute with 1 mL SW for injection and gently swirl to mix. Dose should be given within 6 hr of mixing. Volumes >1 mL should be given as divided dose. May see slight increase in incidence of rhinitis, rash, pain, increased LFTs, pharyngitis, cough, wheeze, diarrhea, vomiting, conjunctivitis, and anemia.

pemoline (Cylert)

Indications

(CNS stimulant)

Used in children for treatment of ADHD and narcolepsy.

Administration

Child ≥6 yr:

Initial:	37.5 mg q AM PO; increase in 18.75-mg/24 hr increments q wk
Maintenance:	0.5–3 mg/kg/24 hr (effective range: 56.25–75 mg/24 hr) (max. dose: 112.5 mg/24 hr)

Nursing Implications

Classified as schedule-IV drug by FCS Act. Liver enzyme studies recommended before therapy; if elevated, drug should not be used. Baseline growth indices are plotted on growth grids and monitored while child is taking medication. Obtain periodic reports from caregivers and teachers regarding behavior. May take 3–4 wk for positive changes in child's behavior. Drug can produce dependence and abuse is a potential. May cause insomnia, HA, seizures, anorexia, depression, abdominal pain, movement disorders, and hepatotoxicity. Contraindicated in patients with Tourette's syndrome.

penicillin G (benzathine preparations) (Bicillin L-A)

Indications

(antibiotic; penicillin, very long-acting IM)

Used in treatment of mild to moderate infections, such as group A streptococcal pharyngitis, and to prevent rheumatic fever.

Administration

Group A streptococci:	
Infant/child:	25,000–50,000 U/kg/dose × 1 IM max. dose: 1.2 million U/dose *or*
>1 mo, <27 kg:	600,000 U/dose × 1 IM
≥27 kg–adult:	1.2 million U/dose × 1 IM
Rheumatic fever prophylaxis:	
Infant/child:	25,000–50,000 U/kg IM q3–4wk (max. dose: 1.2 million U/dose)
Adult:	1.2 million U/dose IM q3–4wk *or* 600,000 U/dose IM q2wk
Compatibility:	Sterile H_2O for injection

Nursing Implications

Do not give IV. Side effects similar to those in aqueous penicillin G. Provides sustained levels for 2–4 wk. Not recommended for treatment of congenital syphilis.

penicillin G (potassium and sodium preparations) (Many brands)

Indications

(antibiotic; aqueous penicillin)

Used in treatment of pneumonia, sepsis, group B streptococcal meningitis, syphilis, and gonorrhea.

Administration

Neonate:	
≤7 days, ≤2 kg:	50,000–100,000 U/kg/24 hr ÷ q12h IV/IM
>2 kg:	75,000–150,000 U/kg/24 hr ÷ q8h IV/IM
>7 days, <1.2 kg:	50,000–100,000 U/kg/24 hr ÷ q12h IV/IM
1.2–2 kg:	75,000–150,000 U/kg/24 hr ÷ q8h IV/IM
≥2 kg:	100,000–200,000 U/kg/24 hr ÷ q6h IV/IM
Congenital syphilis:	
≤7 days:	100,000 U/kg/24 hr ÷ q12h IV/IM
>7 days:	150,000 U/kg/24 hr ÷ q8h IV/IM
Group B streptococcal meningitis:	
≤7 days:	250,000–450,000 U/kg/24 hr ÷ q8h IV/IM
>7 days:	450,000 U/kg/24 hr ÷ q6h IV/IM
Infant/child:	100,000–400,000 U/kg/24 hr ÷ q4–6h IV/IM (max. dose: 24 million U/24 hr)
Adult:	4–24 million U/24 hr ÷ q4–6h IV/IM
IV dilution:	100,000–500,000 U/mL over 15–60 min 50,000 U/mL over 15–30 min recommended for neonates/infants
Compatibility:	D_5W, NS, LR

Nursing Implications

Dose adjustment in renal impairment. Can cause anaphylaxis, hemolytic anemia, and urticaria.

penicillin G (procaine preparations) (Wycillin, Crysticillin A.S.)

Indications

(antibiotic; penicillin, long-acting IM)

Used to treat moderately severe infections and congenital syphilis.

Administration

Neonate:	50,000 U/kg/24 hr q.d. IM
Congenital syphilis:	50,000 U/kg/24 hr q.d. IM × 10 days
Infant/Child:	25,000–50,000 U/kg/24 hr ÷ q12–24h IM (max. dose: 4.8 million U/24 hr)
Adult:	0.6–4.8 million U/24 hr ÷ q12–24h IM
Compatibility:	Sterile H_2O for injection

Nursing Implications

Do not give IV. May cause pain at IM injection site. If >1 day of treatment for congenital syphilis is missed, whole course should be restarted. Side effects similar to those in aqueous penicillin G, plus CNS stimulation and seizures.

penicillin V potassium (Pen•Vee K, V-Cillin K, and others)

Indications

(antibiotic; penicillin)

Used to treat mild to moderately severe bacterial infections of the upper respiratory tract, skin, and urinary tract; to treat group A streptococcal pharyngitis; and for prophylaxis of pneumococcal infections and rheumatic fever.

Administration

Child:	25–50 mg/kg/24 hr ÷ q6–8h PO (max. dose: 3 g/24 hr)
Adult:	250–500 mg/dose q6–8h PO
Acute group A streptococcal pharyngitis:	
Child:	250 mg b.i.d.–t.i.d. PO × 10 days
Adolescent/adult:	500 mg b.i.d.–t.i.d. PO × 10 days
Secondary rheumatic fever/ pneumococcal prophylaxis:	
≤5 yr:	125 mg b.i.d. PO
>5 yr:	250 mg b.i.d. PO

Nursing Implications

Better GI absorption than penicillin G. Can cause rash, nausea, vomiting, diarrhea, and black hairy tongue. Best taken 1 hr before or 2 hr after meals, but can be taken with meals to decrease GI upset.

phenobarbital (Luminal, Solfoton, and others)

Indications

(barbiturate)

Used as anticonvulsant in grand mal, partial, and febrile seizures. Also used for sedation and for prevention and treatment of neonatal hyperbilirubinemia.

Administration

Sedation:	
Child:	6 mg/kg/24 hr ÷ t.i.d. PO

Adult:	30–120 mg/24 hr PO ÷ b.i.d.–t.i.d.
Preoperative sedation:	
Child:	1–3 mg/kg/dose IV/IM/PO 60–90 min before procedure
Status epilepticus:	
Loading dose IV:	
Neonate/infant/child:	15–20 mg/kg in single or divided dose; may give additional 5-mg/kg doses q15–30 min to max. dose of 30 mg/kg
Maintenance dose PO/IV:	
Neonate:	3–5 mg/kg/24 hr ÷ q.d.–b.i.d.
Infant:	5–6 mg/kg/24 hr ÷ q.d.–b.i.d.
1–5 yr:	6–8 mg/kg/24 hr ÷ q.d.–b.i.d.
6–12 yr:	4–6 mg/kg/24 hr ÷ q.d.–b.i.d.
>12 yr:	1–3 mg/kg/24 hr ÷ q.d.–b.i.d.
Hyperbilirubinemia:	
<12 yr:	3–8 mg/kg/24 hr ÷ q.d.–b.i.d.
IV dilution:	
Direct IV:	1 mg/kg/min (max. dose: 30 mg/min for infant/child; 60 mg/min for adult >60 kg)
Infusion:	2 mg/kg/min over 20–30 min
Compatibility:	D_5W, NS, LR, $D_{10}W$

Nursing Implications

IV administration may cause respiratory arrest or hypotension. Side effects include drowsiness, cognitive impairment, ataxia, hypotension, hepatitis, rash, respiratory depression, and apnea. Can also cause hyperactivity, irritability, and insomnia as paradoxical reaction in children. Therapeutic levels: 15–40 mg/L.

phenytoin (Dilantin)

Indications

(anticonvulsant; class 1b antiarrhythmic)

Used in treatment and prevention of grand mal and complex partial seizures. Also used to treat ventricular arrhythmias associated with digitalis intoxication, prolonged Q-T interval, and surgical repair of congenital heart diseases.

Administration

Status epilepticus:	
Loading dose (all ages):	15–20 mg/kg/dose IV (max. dose: 1,500 mg/24 hr)

Maintenance for seizure disorders:	
Neonate:	5–8 mg/kg/24 hr ÷ q8–12h PO/IV
Infant/child:	Start 5 mg/kg/24 hr ÷ b.i.d.–t.i.d. PO/IV
Usual ranges:	
6 mo–3 yr:	8–10 mg/kg/24 hr b.i.d.–t.i.d. PO/IV
4–6 yr:	7.5–9 mg/kg/24 hr b.i.d.–t.i.d. PO/IV
7–9 yr:	7–8 mg/kg/24 hr b.i.d.–t.i.d. PO/IV
10–16 yr:	6–7 mg/kg/24 hr b.i.d.–t.i.d. PO/IV
Adult:	Start with 100 mg/dose q8h PO/IV
Range:	300–600 mg/24 hr *or* 6–7 mg/kg/24 hr ÷ q8–24h PO/IV
Anti-arrhythmia:	
Loading dose (all ages):	1.25 mg/kg q5min IV up to total of 15 mg/kg
Maintenance:	
Child:	5–10 mg/kg/24 hr ÷ q12h PO/IV
Adult:	250 mg q.i.d. PO × 1 day, then 250 mg q12h × 2 days, then 300–400 mg/24 hr ÷ q6–24h
IV dilution:	
Direct IV:	Not to exceed 0.5 mg/kg/min in neonates, 1–3 mg/kg/min in others for max. rate of 50 mg/min. Flush with NS.
Intermittent IV:	Dilute with NS to <6 mg/mL
Compatibility:	NS only

Nursing Implications

Crystallizes with dextrose. Contraindicated in patients with heart block or sinus bradycardia. IM route not recommended. Assess for irritation and necrosis with IV use. Therapeutic levels for seizure disorders: 10–20 mg/L. Side effects include gingival hyperplasia, hirsutism, dermatitis, blood dyscrasias, ataxia, Stevens-Johnson syndrome, lymphadenopathy, liver damage, and nystagmus. Many drug interactions, so check insert or with pharmacist.

piperacillin (Pipracil)

Indications

(antibiotic; extended spectrum penicillin)

Used in treatment of serious infections of skin, bone, joint, respiratory tract, and urinary tract. Often used for patients with CF. Also used to treat intraabdominal and gynecologic infections. Primary use is in treatment of serious carbenicillin- or ticarcillin-resistant *Pseudomonas aeruginosa* infections.

Administration

Neonate:	
≤7 days, ≤36 wk gestation:	150 mg/kg/24 hr ÷ q12h IV
>36 wk gestation:	225 mg/kg/24 hr ÷ q8h IV
>7 days, ≤36 wk gestation:	225 mg/kg/24 hr ÷ q8h IV
>36 wk gestation:	300 mg/kg/24 hr ÷ q6h IV
Infant/child:	200–300 mg/kg/24 hr ÷ 4–6h IV/IM (max. dose: 24 g/24 hr)
CF:	300–600 mg/kg/24 hr ÷ q4–6h IV/IM (max. dose: 24 g/24 hr)
Adult:	2–4 g/dose q4–6h IV *or* 1–2 g/dose q6h IM (max. dose: 24 g/24 hr)
IV dilution:	
Direct IV:	200 mg/mL over 3–5 min
Intermittent IV:	≤20 mg/mL over 30–60 min
Compatibility:	D_5W, NS, LR

Nursing Implications

May cause seizures, myoclonus, and fever. Assess IV site for irritation and phlebitis. Administer IM dose deep in a large muscle. If child is also receiving IV aminoglycosides, separate infusions by ≥2 hr.

potassium chloride (Many brands)

Indications

(KCl supplements)
Used to correct or prevent potassium deficiency.

Administration

Normal daily requirements:	
Neonate/infant:	2–6 mEq/kg/24 hr IV/PO
Child:	2–3 mEq/kg/24 hr IV/PO
Adult:	40–80 mEq/24 hr IV/PO
Hypokalemia:	
Child:	1–4 mEq/kg/24 hr ÷ b.i.d.–q.i.d. PO 0.5–1 mEq/dose given as infusion of 0.5 mEq/kg/hr × 1–2 hr (max. IV infusion rate: 1 mEq/kg/hr in critical situations)
Adult:	40–100 mEq/24 hr ÷ b.i.d.–q.i.d. PO 10–20 mEq/dose to infuse over 2–3 hr (max. IV infusion rate: 40 mEq/hr)

IV dilution:	Max. peripheral IV solution concentration: 40 mEq/L Max. concentration for CVL: 150–200 mEq/L *Do not give IV push.*
Compatibility:	D_5W, NS, LR

Nursing Implications

Rapid IV infusion can cause arrhythmias. PO administration may cause GI disturbance and ulceration. Oral liquid should be diluted in water or juice. Monitor potassium levels.

prednisone (Deltasone and others)

Indications

(corticosteroid)

Used in management of adrenocortical insufficiency and for anti-inflammatory and immunosuppressant effects.

Administration

Anti-inflammatory/ immunosuppressive:	0.5–2 mg/kg/24 hr ÷ q.d.–b.i.d. PO
Acute asthma:	2 mg/kg/24 hr q.d.–b.i.d. PO × 5 days (max. dose: 80 mg/24 hr)
Nephrotic syndrome:	
Initial:	2 mg/kg/24 hr PO (max. dose: 80 mg/24 hr)

Nursing Implications

Doses must be tapered gradually to discontinue unless used ≤5 days. Further doses in nephrotic syndrome are individualized by nephrologist. Side effects include mood changes, seizures, hyperglycemia, diarrhea, nausea, and GI bleeding. Patients can have cushingoid effects and cataracts with prolonged use. Barbiturates, carbamazepine, phenytoin, rifampin, and INH may reduce effects of prednisone, whereas estrogens may enhance effects. Administer after meals or with food to decrease GI upset.

promethazine (Phenergan, Provigan, and others)

Indications

(antihistamine; antiemetic; phenothiazine derivative)

Used in symptomatic treatment of allergic conditions and motion sickness, as preoperative sedative, and for prevention and treatment of nausea and vomiting.

Administration

Antihistaminic:	
Child:	0.1 mg/kg/dose q6h PO and 0.5 mg/kg/dose q h.s. p.r.n. PO
Adult:	12.5 mg t.i.d. PO and 25 mg q h.s. PO
Sedation:	
Child:	0.5–1.1 mg/kg/dose q6h p.r.n. PO/PR/IV/IM
Adult:	25–50 mg/dose q4–6h p.r.n. PO/PR/IV/IM
Nausea and vomiting:	
Child:	0.25–1 mg/kg/dose q4–6h p.r.n. PO/PR/IV/IM
Adult:	12.5–25 mg q4–6h p.r.n. PO/PR/IV/IM
Motion sickness:	First dose 0.5–1 hr before departure
Child:	0.5 mg/kg/dose q12h p.r.n. PO
Adult:	25 mg b.i.d. p.r.n. PO
IV dilution:	Undiluted 25 mg/mL no faster than 25 mg/min
Compatibility:	D_5W, NS, LR, $D_{10}W$

Nursing Implications

Observe for excessive sedation. Monitor BP, pulse, and respirations with IV use. IM administration preferred. Administer with food or milk to decrease GI distress. May cause profound sedation, blurred vision, and dystonic reactions.

ranitidine (Zantac)

Indications

(histamine-2 antagonist)

Used in prevention and treatment of duodenal ulcers and in management of GE reflux.

Administration

Neonate:	2–4 mg/kg/24 hr ÷ q8–12h PO 2 mg/kg/24 hr ÷ q6–8h IV
Infant/child:	4–5 mg/kg/24 hr ÷ q8–12h PO (max. dose: 6 mg/kg/24 hr) 2–4 mg/kg/24 hr ÷ q6–8h IV/IM
Adult:	150 mg/dose b.i.d. *or* 300 mg/dose q h.s. PO 50 mg/dose q6–8h IV/IM (max. dose: 400 mg/24 hr)
Continuous infusion (all ages):	Administer daily IV dose over 24 hr

IV dilution:

Direct IV:	2.5 mg/mL over 5 min
Intermittent infusion (preferred):	0.5 mg/mL over 15–30 min

Compatibility: D_5W, NS, LR, $D_{10}W$

Nursing Implications

Rapid infusion can cause bradycardia, tachycardia, or premature ventricular contractions. Can be added to total parenteral nutrition. Can cause headache, GI disturbances, malaise, insomnia, sedation, arthralgia, and hepatotoxicity. Antacids decrease absorption.

respiratory syncytial virus immune globulin intravenous (RSV-IGIV) (RespiGam)

Indications

(immune globulin, RSV, high titer)

Used to prevent RSV infection in infants at risk. Broadly indicated for use in children <2 yr old with bronchopulmonary dysplasia (BPD) or history of prematurity (<35 weeks' gestation). For current specific-use recommendations, see newest edition of American Academy of Pediatrics (AAP) Red Book (AAP, 2000).

Administration

Child <2 yr:	750 mg/kg/dose IV q mo during RSV season
IV infusion:	1.5 mL/kg/hr × 15 min, then 3 mL/kg/hr × 15 min, then 6 mL/kg/hr to end of infusion (max. rate: 6 mL/kg/hr)

Nursing Implications

Should not be used in patients with cyanotic heart disease. Contraindicated in immunoglobulin A deficiency. Use with caution in patients with fluid restrictions. Common side effects include fever, respiratory distress, vomiting, and wheezing. Monitor HR, BP, and respiratory rate during administration. Measles-mumps-rubella and varicella-zoster vaccines should be deferred 9–10 mo after last dose of RSV-IGIV. RSV season typically November through April.

spironolactone (Aldactone)

Indications

(diuretic, potassium sparing)

Used in management of edema, hypertension, and primary hyperaldosteronism and in treatment of hirsutism.

Administration

Diuretic:

Child:	1–3.3 mg/kg/24 hr ÷ b.i.d.–q.i.d. PO
Adult:	25–200 mg/24 hr ÷ b.i.d.–q.i.d. PO (max. dose: 200 mg/24 hr)

Primary aldosteronism:

Child:	125–325 mg/m^2/24 hr b.i.d.–q.i.d. PO
Adult:	400 mg q.d. PO × 4 days or 3–4 wk, then 100–400 mg q.d. maintenance

Nursing Implications

Administer with food. Contraindicated in acute renal failure. May cause hyperkalemia, GI distress, rash, and gynecomastia. Potassium levels should be monitored.

sulfisoxazole (Gantrisin)

Indications

(antibiotic; sulfonamide derivative)

Used in treatment of UTIs, OM, and RF and for meningococcus prophylaxis.

Administration

Children ≥2 mo:	
Initial:	75 mg/kg/dose PO × 1
Maintenance:	120–150 mg/kg/24 hr ÷ q4–6h PO (max. dose: 6 g/24 hr)
Adult:	
Initial:	2–4 g × 1
Maintenance:	4–8 g/24 hr ÷ q4–6h PO (max. dose: 8 g/24 hr)
OM prophylaxis:	50 mg/kg/dose q h.s. PO
RF prophylaxis:	
<27 kg:	500 mg q.d. PO
≥27 kg:	100 mg q.d. PO
Meningococcus prophylaxis:	
<1 yr:	500 mg q.d. PO × 2 days
1–12 yr:	500 mg b.i.d. PO × 2 days
>12 yr:	1,000 mg b.i.d. PO × 2 days
Ophthalmic solution:	1–2 gtt. q1–4h

Nursing Implications

Give on empty stomach. Do not use in infants <2 mo of age. Contraindicated in urinary obstruction. Use with caution in renal or liver disease or G6PD deficiency. Maintain adequate fluid intake. Can cause HA, fever, rash, Stevens-Johnson syndrome, nausea, vomiting, and blood dyscrasias.

ticarcillin (Ticar)

Indications

(antibiotic; extended-spectrum penicillin)

Used in treatment of serious infections of skin, bone, joints, and urinary tract; acute and chronic respiratory tract infections; and septicemia. Often used to treat lung infections in children with CF.

Administration

Neonates:	
≤7 days, <2 kg:	150 mg/kg/24 hr ÷ q12h IV/IM
≥2 kg:	225 mg/kg/24 hr ÷ q8h IV/IM
>7 days, <1.2 kg:	150 mg/kg/24 hr ÷ q12h IV/IM
1.2–2 kg:	225 mg/kg/24 hr ÷ q8h IV/IM
>2 kg:	300 mg/kg/24 hr ÷ q6–8h IV/IM
Infant/child:	200–300 mg/kg/24 hr ÷ q4–6h IV/IM (max. dose: 24 g/24 hr)
Adult:	1–4 g/dose q4-6h IV/IM
Uncomplicated UTIs:	
Child:	50–100 mg/kg/24 hr ÷ q6–8h IV/IM
Adult:	1 g/dose q6h IV/IM
CF:	300–600 mg/kg/24 hr ÷ q4–6h IV/IM (max. dose: 24 g/24 hr)
IV dilution:	100 mg/mL over 30–120 min; ≤50 mg/mL preferred
Compatibility:	D_5W, NS, LR

Nursing Implications

May cause decreased platelet aggregation, hypocalcemia, hypokalemia, hypernatremia, rash, hematuria, and increased aspartate aminotransferase. If child also receiving IV aminoglycosides, separate infusions by ≥2 hr.

ticarcillin/clavulanate (Timentin)

Indications

(antibiotic; extended-spectrum penicillin with β-lactamase inhibitor)

Same as ticarcillin except has β-lactamase inhibitor that broadens spectrum.

Administration

Doses based on ticarcillin; see ticarcillin (max. dose: 18–24 g/24 hr)

Nursing Implications

Same as ticarcillin.

tobramycin (Tobrex, Nebcin, TOBI, and others)

Indications

(antibiotic; aminoglycoside)

Used in treatment of serious gram-negative and staphylococcal infections when penicillin is contraindicated or gentamicin resistance has occurred. Also effective against *P. aeruginosa*. Used topically to treat ophthalmic infections and as inhalation therapy for management of CF patients with *P. aeruginosa*.

Administration

Neonate:	Dose depends on postconceptual and postnatal age and weight; consult pharmacology text
Child:	6–7.5 mg/kg/24 hr ÷ q8h IV/IM
CF:	7.5–10 mg/kg/24 hr ÷ q8h IV
Adult:	3–6 mg/kg/24 hr ÷ q8h IV/IM
Ophthalmic:	Apply thin ribbon of ointment to affected eye b.i.d.–t.i.d. *or* 1–2 gtt. of solution q4h
CF prophylaxis therapy (TOBI):	
≥6 yr–adult:	300 mg q12h in repeated cycles of 28 days on and 28 days off drug
IV dilution:	≤10 mg/mL over 30–60 min *or* direct injection over 15 min
Compatibility:	D_5W, NS

Nursing Implications

Therapeutic levels: peak: 6–10 mg/L (8–10 mg/L in pulmonary infections, neutropenia, and severe sepsis); trough: <2 mg/L. Can cause ototoxicity (effects synergistic with furosemide) and nephrotoxicity. Can also cause HA, rash, nausea, vomiting, weakness, and elevated liver enzymes.

When giving TOBI with other inhaled medicines, give it last. Separate IV administration from other antibiotics by ≥1 hr.

valproic acid/valproate sodium (Depakene, Depacon)

Indications

(anticonvulsant)

Used in management of simple and complex partial seizures, absence seizures, mixed seizure types, and myoclonic and grand mal seizures.

Administration

Initial:	10–15 mg/kg/24 hr ÷ q.d.–t.i.d. PO
Increment:	5–10 mg/kg/24 hr q wk (max. dose: 60 mg/kg/24 hr)
Maintenance:	30–60 mg/kg/24 hr ÷ b.i.d.–t.i.d. PO
IV:	Use same dose as PO ÷ q6h; convert back to PO as soon as possible
PR:	Use syrup diluted 1:1 with water; given PR as retention enema
Load:	20 mg/kg/dose
Maintenance:	10–15 mg/kg/dose q8h
IV dilution:	Dilute with ≥50 mL over 60 min (max. rate: 20 mg/min)
Compatibility:	D_5W, NS, LR

Nursing Implications

Contraindicated in hepatic disease. Can cause GI, blood, CNS, and liver toxicity; weight gain; transient alopecia; pancreatitis; nausea; vomiting; sedation; HA; and rash. Increases phenytoin, diazepam, and phenobarbital levels. Phenytoin, phenobarbital, and carbamazepine decrease valproic acid levels. Do not give syrup with carbonated beverages. Do not give tablet with milk. Therapeutic levels: 50–100 mg/L.

vancomycin (Vancocin and others)

Indications

(antibiotic)

Used in treatment of life-threatening infections such as endocarditis, meningitis, and osteomyelitis; in documented or suspected methicillin-resistant *Staphylococcus aureus*; and for infections associated with central lines, ventriculoperitoneal shunts, hemodialysis shunts, vascular grafts, and prosthetic heart valves. Used orally to treat staphylococcal enterocolitis or antibiotic-associated pseudomembranous colitis produced by *Clostridium difficile*.

Administration

Neonate:

<7 days, <1.2 kg:	15 mg/kg/dose q24h IV
1.2–2 kg:	10–15 mg/kg/dose q12–18h IV

>2 kg:	10–15 mg/kg/dose q8–12h IV
≥7 days, <1.2 kg:	15 mg/kg/dose q24h IV
1.2–2 kg:	10–15 mg/kg/dose q8–12h IV
>2 kg:	15–20 mg/kg/dose q8h IV
Infant/child:	
CNS infection:	60 mg/kg/24 hr ÷ q6h IV
Other:	40 mg/kg/24 hr ÷ q6–8h IV (max. dose: 1 g/dose)
Adult:	2 g/24 hr ÷ q6–12h IV
C. difficile colitis:	
Child:	40–50 mg/kg/24 hr ÷ q6h PO × 7–10 days (max. dose: 500 mg/24 hr)
Adult:	125 mg/dose q6h PO × 7–10 days
IV dilution:	5 mg/mL over 60 min
Compatibility:	D_5W, NS, LR, $D_{10}W$

Nursing Implications

"Red man syndrome" (red flushing of neck and head with intense pruritus) with too rapid infusion. May need to increase infusion time to 120 min. Can also cause tachycardia, hypotension, chills, and nausea. Ototoxicity and nephrotoxicity may occur and may be exacerbated with concurrent aminoglycoside use. Therapeutic levels: peak: 25–40 mg/L; trough: <10 mg/L. Controversial whether levels need to be monitored.

DRUG ADMINISTRATION

IV Fluid Dilution and Rate Calculations

Determining Proper Dilution

Recommended dilution of a particular drug is 10 mg/mL.
Patient's dose is 500 mg IV q6h.

To determine the amount of fluid needed to dilute a particular drug, use the following equation:

$$\frac{10\text{ mg}}{1\text{ mL}} = \frac{500\text{ mg}}{x\text{ mL}}\ \text{(Cross multiply)}$$

$$10x = 500$$

$$x = 50\text{ mL}$$

So you will dilute 500 mg in 50 mL to get proper concentration of 10 mg/mL.

Determining Proper Rate

Many IV pumps can be set for volume and time, so this step may not be necessary.

$$\frac{\text{volume to be infused} \times \text{drip factor}}{\text{time (min)}} = \text{drops (gtt.)/min}$$

Example: We want to dilute the aforementioned drug in 50 mL and give over 30 min. Drip factor in pediatric clients is usually 60 because of use of microdrips.

$$\frac{50 \text{ mL} \times 60}{30 \text{ min}} = \frac{3{,}000}{30}$$

= 100 gtt./min or with drip factor of 60 drops/mL, is also 30 min. 100 mL/hr

Syringe pumps can be set for amount to be infused and for time.

Safe Drug Calculations

Determine child's weight in kilograms.

Example: Child weighs 22 pounds.

$$22 \text{ pounds} \div 2.2 \text{ pounds/kg} = 10 \text{ kg}$$

Recommended safe dose is 200–400 mg/kg/24 hr q6h.

Calculate 200 mg × 10 kg and 400 mg × 10 kg to get safe range for 24 hr. Safe range 2,000–4,000 mg/24 hr. Divide by 4 to get safe range for each dose given q6h. Safe dose range 500–1,000 mg/dose.

The aforementioned drug comes in a solution of 1,000 mg/mL. We want to give a dose of 500 mg. To calculate amount to draw up, use the following equation:

$$\frac{1{,}000 \text{ mg}}{1 \text{ mL}} = \frac{500 \text{ mg}}{x \text{ mL}} \text{ (Cross multiply)}$$

$$1{,}000x = 500$$

$$x = 0.5 \text{ mL}$$

Preparation for Drug Administration

General Guidelines

- Start with clean area.
- Verify MD/APRN medication order.
- Obtain proper drug and proper strength.
- Assemble needed equipment.

- Draw up medication or check unit dose.
- Make sure you have necessary supplies (e.g., alcohol swab, bandages, proper needle for IV system, label, nipple, syringe, cup, drink) before entering client's room.
- Take med sheet or card to compare with client's identification band.
- Know how client has taken and tolerated medications previously (e.g., can client swallow pills? can client tolerate volume?)
- Do not give medications in playroom. It is a safe area. Take child out of playroom to administer any medication.
- Be truthful; let child know what to expect. Explain child and caregiver roles. Try not to let caregiver threaten child. Encourage caregivers to comfort only.

Infants	Need TLC before and after.
Toddlers	Need immediate preparation. Do not offer unreal choices. Allow caregiver to help with oral medications.
Preschool children	Need to know what they are expected to do. Let them handle equipment. A bandage is very important for body integrity.
School-aged children	Need explanation of their role and choices when possible. Longer preparation time needed for invasive procedures.
Adolescents	Generally want more information. Privacy is important. Preserve "tough" image. Recognize need for independence. Allow client choices (e.g., site), if appropriate.

Administration

Five Rights

Right drug
Right dose
Right time
Right route
Right client

Oral Medications

Crush tablets and mix with small amount of hot water and then syrup. Do not mix in large volumes or add to infant's bottle. Be aware of taste. Syrups are sweet, elixirs are bitter. Use cup, spoon, syringe, nipple (with syrups only) as appropriate for client. Give slowly. If using syringe, place it halfway back at side of tongue. Remember normal tongue thrust present until 4–5 mo.

Intramuscular (IM)

Site	Comment
Vastus lateralis	Most medications
Ventro gluteal	Not until 3 yr; check hospital policy
Gluteus maximus	Must be walking for ≥1 yr; any medication
Deltoid	Less invasive; usually not used until 3 yr; use with nonirritating medications

Age	Amount
Birth–3 yr	1 mL
3–6 yr	1.5 mL
6–15 yr	1.5–2 mL
Adult	2–3 mL

Age	Needle size
Birth–4 mo	5/8 inch
4 mo–10 yr	1 inch
10 yr–adult	$1\frac{1}{2}$ inch

Use smallest gauge needle possible; larger gauges may be needed for viscous medications and to prevent bending.

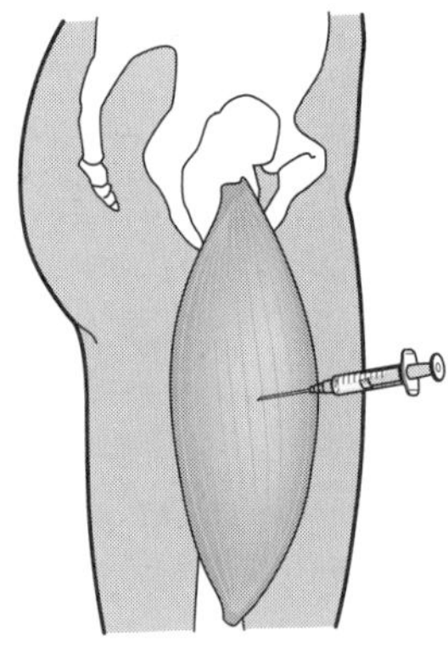

Vastus lateralis

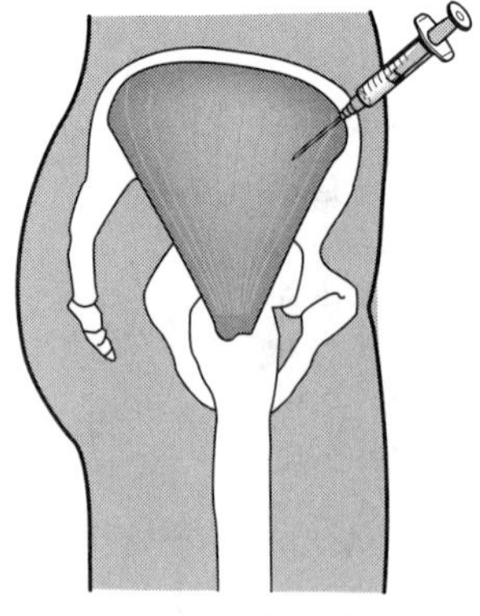

Ventrogluteal

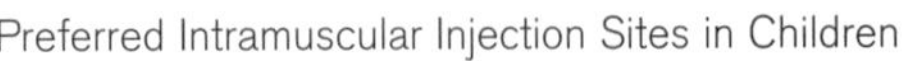

Preferred Intramuscular Injection Sites in Children

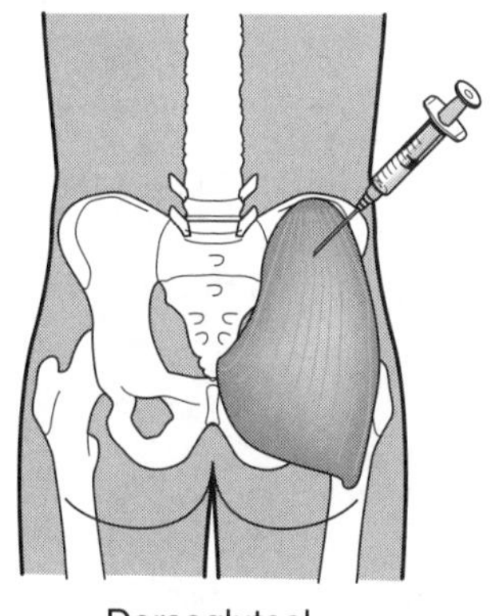

Dorsogluteal

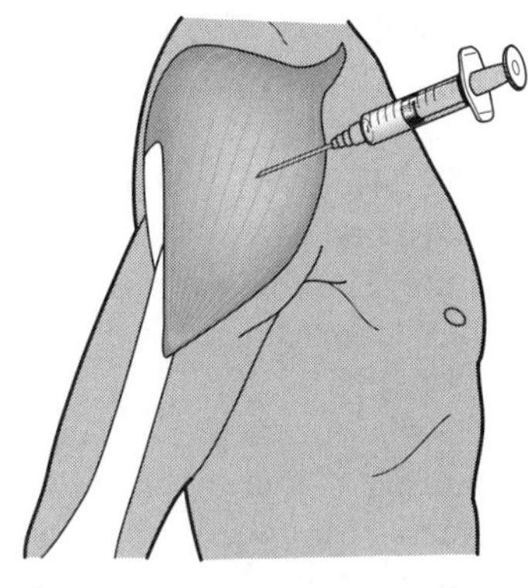

Deltoid

Preferred Intramuscular Injection Sites in Children

Subcutaneous (SC)

Sites	Same as IM
Amount	0.5 mL
Needle size	5/8–1 inch

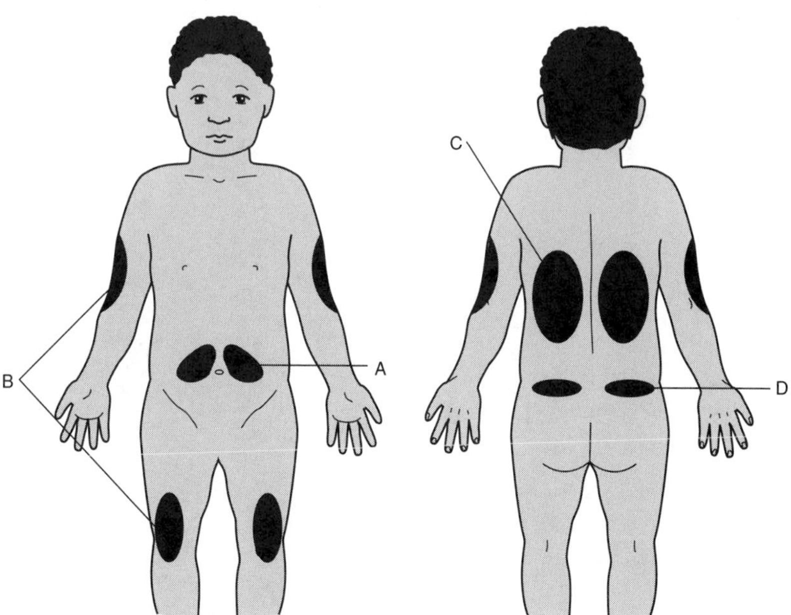

Subcutaneous Injection Sites: A. Abdomen; B. Lateral and Anterior Aspects of Upper Arm and Thigh; C. Scapular Area of Back; D. Upper Ventrodorsal Gluteal Area

Intravenous (IV)

Follow guidelines for proper dilution and time.

Check IV site for patency before and during infusion.

Check to be sure site and needle size adequate for volume to be administered.

Flush IV tubing at same rate as medication administration to make sure all medication has been administered.

Rectal

Is invasive to most ages. Have preschoolers "pant like a puppy dog" to relax sphincter. May need to hold buttock cheeks together to prevent expelling. If you need to divide suppository to get correct dose, do so lengthwise to allow for easier insertion and to get better distribution of medication.

Nasogastric (NG)/Gastrostomy Tube (GT)

Check for placement before administering medications. Be sure to crush pills well and flush with water to prevent clogging tube.

Topical

Apply thin layer because of increased skin permeability.

Diaper can act as occlusive dressing and cause increased absorption of medication.

Eye

Put drops in inner canthus. Put ointment in lower lid. Tell child that ointment will blur vision. If child will not cooperate, place drops in inner canthus and hold head still so he or she cannot turn to the side. When child opens his or her eyes to see why you have not gone away, medication will go into the eyes. Apply pressure to the puncta at inner aspect of lower lid for 1 min to help prevent medication from going into nasopharynx.

Ear

In children <3 yr, pull pinnae down and back to straighten ear canal. If >3 yr, pull pinnae up and back. Try to keep child on his or her side for 1 min after administration if possible. Make sure medication is warmed to at least room temperature.

Nasal

Tip head back and keep back for 1 min after administration of drops if possible to prevent strangling sensation of medication running into the posterior pharynx. Remember to sit child up for administration of nasal sprays so they will properly aerosolize.

Immunization Schedule

Recommended Childhood Immunization Schedule United States, January-December 2001

Vaccines[1] are listed under routinely recommended ages. Bars indicate range of recommended ages for immunization. Any dose not given at the recommended age should be given as a "catch-up" immunization at any subsequent visit when indicated and feasible. Ovals indicate vaccines to be given if previously recommended doses were missed or given earlier than the recommended minimum age.

Age ▶ Vaccines ▼	Birth	1 mo	2 mos	4 mos	6 mos	12 mos	15 mos	18 mos	24 mos	4-6 yrs	11-12 yrs	14-16 yrs
Hepatitis B[2]		Hep B #1										
			Hep B # 2			Hep B # 3					Hep B[2]	
Diphtheria, Tetanus, Pertussis[3]			DTaP	DTaP	DTaP			DTaP[3]		DTaP	Td	
H. influenzae type b[4]			Hib	Hib	Hib	Hib						
Inactivated Polio[5]			IPV	IPV		IPV[5]				IPV[5]		
Pneumococcal Conjugate[6]			PCV	PCV	PCV	PCV						
Measles, Mumps, Rubella[7]						MMR				MMR[7]	MMR[7]	
Varicella[8]							Var				Var[8]	
Hepatitis A[9]											Hep A—in selected areas[9]	

Approved by the Advisory Committee on Immunization Practices (ACIP), the American Academy of Pediatrics (AAP), and the American Academy of Family Physicians (AAFP).

1. This schedule indicates the recommended ages for routine administration of currently licensed childhood vaccines, as of 11/1/00, for children through 18 years of age. Additional vaccines may be licensed and recommended during the year. Licensed combination vaccines may be used whenever any components of the combination are indicated and its other components are not contraindicated. Providers should consult the manufacturers' package inserts for detailed recommendations.
2. *Infants born to HBsAg-negative mothers* should receive the 1st dose of hepatitis B (Hep B) vaccine by age 2 months. The 2nd dose should be at least one month after the 1st dose. The 3rd dose should be administered at least 4 months after the 1st dose and at least 2 months after the 2nd dose, but not before 6 months of age for infants.
   Infants born to HBsAg-positive mothers should receive hepatitis B vaccine and 0.5 mL hepatitis B immune globulin (HBIG) within 12 hours of birth at separate sites. The 2nd dose is recommended at 1-2 months of age and the 3rd dose at 6 months of age.
   Infants born to mothers whose HBsAg status is unknown should receive hepatitis B vaccine within 12 hours of birth. Maternal blood should be drawn at the time of delivery to determine the mother's HBsAg status; if the HBsAg test is positive, the infant should receive HBIG as soon as possible (no later than 1 week of age).
   All children and adolescents who have not been immunized against hepatitis B should begin the series during any visit. Special efforts should be made to immunize children who were born in or whose parents were born in areas of the world with moderate or high endemicity of hepatitis B virus infection.
3. The 4th dose of DTaP (diphtheria and tetanus toxoids and acellular pertussis vaccine) may be administered as early as 12 months of age, provided 6 months have elapsed since the 3rd dose and the child is unlikely to return at age 15-18 months. Td (tetanus and diphtheria toxoids) is recommended at 11-12 years of age if at least 5 years have elapsed since the last dose of DTP, DTaP, or DT. Subsequent routine Td boosters are recommended every 10 years.
4. Three *Haemophilus influenzae* type b (Hib) conjugate vaccines are licensed for infant use. If PRP-OMP (PedvaxHIB® or ComVax® [Merck]) is administered at 2 and 4 months of age, a dose at 6 months is not required. Because clinical studies in infants have demonstrated that using some combination products may induce a lower immune response to the Hib vaccine component, DTaP/Hib combination products should not be used for primary immunization in infants at 2, 4, or 6 months of age, unless FDA-approved for these ages.
5. An all-IPV schedule is recommended for routine childhood polio vaccination in the United States. All children should receive four doses of IPV at 2 months, 4 months, 6-18 months, and 4-6 years of age. Oral polio vaccine (OPV) should be used only in selected circumstances. (See MMWR May 19,2000/49(RR-5);1-22).
6. The heptavalent conjugate pneumococcal vaccine (PCV) is recommended for all children 2-23 months of age. It also is recommended for certain children 24-59 months of age. (See MMWR Oct. 6, 2000/49(RR-9);1-35).
7. The 2nd dose of measles, mumps, and rubella (MMR) vaccine is recommended routinely at 4-6 years of age but may be administered during any visit, provided at least 4 weeks have elapsed since receipt of the 1st dose and that both doses are administered beginning at or after 12 months of age. Those who have not previously received the second dose should complete the schedule by the 11-12 year old visit.
8. Varicella (Var) vaccine is recommended at any visit on or after the first birthday for susceptible children, i.e. those who lack a reliable history of chickenpox (as judged by a health care provider) and who have not been immunized. Susceptible persons 13 years of age or older should receive 2 doses, given at least 4 weeks apart.
9. Hepatitis A (Hep A) is shaded to indicate its recommended use in selected states and/or regions, and for certain high risk groups; consult your local public health authority. (See MMWR Oct. 1, 1999/48(RR-12); 1-37).

For additional information about the vaccines listed above, please visit the National Immunization Program Home Page at http://www.cdc.gov/nip/ or call the National Immunization Hotline at 800-232-2522 (English) or 800-232-0233 (Spanish).

Recommended Childhood Immunization Schedule, United States, January–December 2001. From Centers of Disease Control and Prevention.

PEDIATRIC RESUSCITATION DRUGS

You must know (or be able to estimate) the weight of the child because all drug dosages and fluid calculations depend on weight.

WEIGHT PER AGE ESTIMATES

Age	Weight in kg
6 mo	7
1 yr	10
2–3 yr	12–14
3–4 yr	14–16
5–6 yr	18–20
7–8 yr	22–24
9–10 yr	28–34
11–12 yr	40–45
13–14 yr	47–50

When administering resuscitation drugs during a code, use saline flush between all medication doses to prevent drug interactions. All drugs, dosages, administration times, and routes of administration are to be documented accurately. Most facilities have flowsheets for this purpose. Be sure to be familiar with your institution's policies and procedures.

Efforts have been made to ensure drug dosage information herein is accurate and reflects acceptable standards at the time of publication. However, changes in treatment and drug therapy continually occur. Therefore, readers are advised to check product information included with each drug to be sure that changes have not been made.

adenosine

(antiarrhythmic)

Indications

Drug of choice in treatment of symptomatic supraventricular tachycardia (SVT).

Administration

0.1–0.2 mg/kg IV or IO pushed rapidly. Maximum single dose is 12 mg. If unsuccessful, repeat once after 3 min, doubling initial dose.

Nursing Implications

Monitor ECG continuously during administration.

atropine sulfate

(anticholinergic; parasympatholytic)

Indications

Used to treat symptomatic bradycardia and to restore normal heart contraction during cardiac arrest. Increases HR and cardiac output by blocking vagal stimulation in the heart.

Administration

0.02 mg/kg/dose, with minimum dose of 0.1 mg and maximum initial dose of 1.0 mg for an adolescent and 0.5 mg for a small child; give by slow IV. Repeat q5min to maximum total dose of 1 mg in children and 2 mg in adolescents. May be given IV, IO, or ET. Incompatible with sodium bicarbonate and epinephrine.

Nursing Implications

Effect on HR in 2–4 min. Continuous monitoring of vital signs necessary.

bretylium tosylate

(antiarrhythmic)

Indications

Used in prevention and treatment of ventricular fibrillation (V fib) or hemodynamically unstable ventricular tachycardia (V tach). Used if resistant to defibrillation (or cardioversion) and lidocaine.

Administration

5 mg/kg/dose rapid IV infusion. Compatible with D_5 0.45%NS, D_5 0.9%NS, D_5LR, 0.9%NS, 5% dextrose, LR, 5% sodium bicarbonate, 20% mannitol, calcium chloride in 5% dextrose, and potassium chloride in 5% dextrose.

Nursing Implications

Continuous ECG monitoring necessary. Usually used only if lidocaine not effective.

calcium chloride 10%

(electrolyte; calcium salt)

Indications

Used to maintain normal cardiac contractility after cardiac arrest.

Administration

20–50 mg/kg/dose administered slowly IV. Repeated q10min if needed. Compatible with dextrose and sodium chloride.

Nursing Implications

Continuous ECG monitoring necessary.

dopamine

(adrenergic agonist; vasopressor)

Indications

Used to treat shock and correct hemodynamics. Improves perfusion to vital organs and increases cardiac output and BP.

Administration

2–20 μg/kg/min. Start at 10 μg/kg/min in child with shock and titrate up to 20 μg/kg/min. Dilute 200 or 400 mg in 250–500 mL of 5% dextrose, LR, or sodium chloride.

Nursing Implications

Dosage titrated to hemodynamically desired response. Dopamine most effective in patients who are not hypovolemic.

epinephrine

(adrenergic agonist; sympathomimetic)

Indications

Used in cardiac arrest to treat asystole, bradyarrhythmias, pulseless electrical activity, and V fib. Causes vasoconstriction, increased HR, bronchodilation, and cardiac stimulation.

Administration

0.01 mg/kg IV/IO of 1:10,000 solution. Subsequent IV/IO doses of 0.1 mg/kg of 1:10,000 solution. First ET dose of 0.1 mg/kg of 1:1,000 solution with same subsequent doses. Repeat q3–5min p.r.n. Dosage to be given rapidly. Peak levels reached in 1–2 min following IV dose.

Nursing Implications

Continuous ECG monitoring necessary. Drug disappears from bloodstream rapidly. Urine formation may decrease because of renal vessel constriction.

lidocaine

(antiarrhythmic)

Indications

Used in management of acute ventricular arrythmias. Constant infusion should be used in V tach or V fib that reverts after a lidocaine bolus.

Administration

Single bolus of 1.0 mg/kg slowly IV/IO/ET. May repeat in 10–15 min × 2. For continuous infusion give 20–50 μg/kg/min IV.

Nursing Implications

Only lidocaine hydrochloride without epinephrine should be used IV. Continuous ECG and BP monitoring necessary. If signs of toxicity (e.g., myocardial/circulatory depression; CNS symptoms of drowsiness, disorientation, muscle twitching, seizure) are present, discontinue infusion.

naloxone

(narcotic antagonist)

Indications

Used to reverse effects of narcotic depression, including respiratory depression induced by opioids.

Administration

Children (<20 kg) 0.1 mg/kg/dose IM/IV/SC/ET. Repeat q3–5min p.r.n. Children (>20 kg) 2 mg/dose. Repeat q3–5min p.r.n. Compatible with 0.9% sodium chloride or 5% dextrose.

Nursing Implications

Abrupt reversal of narcotic depression may result in nausea, vomiting, diaphoresis, tachycardia, hypertension, and tremors. Maintain open airway and provide artificial ventilation if needed.

oxygen

Indications

Should be used in any condition of respiratory difficulty as well as in resuscitation.

Administration

Highest available percentage should be used during resuscitation, humidified if possible.

sodium bicarbonate 8.4%

(electrolyte; systemic alkalinizer)

Indications

Used to treat cardiac arrest. Not considered first-line resuscitation drug. Used if continued cardiac arrest with severe acidosis.

Administration

0.5–1.0 mEq/kg over 1–2 min IV/IO. Dilute with SW, NS, or D_5W.

Nursing Implications

Monitor cardiac rhythm carefully during IV administration. Give slowly to prevent hypernatremia, decrease in CSF pressure, and possible intracranial hemorrhage.

DEFIBRILLATION AND SYNCHRONIZED CARDIOVERSION

Paddle Size

Use largest electrode size that allows good chest contact over entire area and good separation between the two electrodes. Recommended diameter for infants is 4.5 cm. Recommended diameter for children is 8.0 cm or 13.0 cm for larger children/adolescents. Electrode gel or cream recommended.

Paddle Placement

Heart should be situated between paddles. Ideal placement is anterior/posterior, but not always practical. Standard placement is one paddle on right upper chest below clavicle with other to left of nipple in anterior axillary line.

Energy Dose

2 J/kg for initial defibrillation. Second and all subsequent defibrillation attempts 4 J/kg. For initial cardioversion dose is 0.5–1.0 J/kg. For second and all subsequent cardioversion attempts use dose of 2.0 J/kg.

CHAPTER 5

ESSENTIAL CLINICAL SKILLS

DETERMINING ENDOTRACHEAL TUBE (ETT), SUCTION CATHETER, AND LARYNGOSCOPE BLADE SIZES

Age	Weight (in kg)	ETT Size	Suction Catheter	Laryngoscope Blade
Newborn	3	3.0–3.5	6 French	1
Infant	5	3.5–4.0	8 French	1
1 yr	10	4.0–4.5	8 French	1½
3 yr	15	4.5–4.0	8 French	2
6 yr	20	5.0–5.5	10 French	2
10 yr	30	6.0–6.5 cuffed	10 French	2
Adolescent	50	7.0–7.5 cuffed	10 French	3
Adult	70	7.5–8.0 cuffed	12–14 French	3

$$\text{Endotracheal tube diameter (mm)} = \frac{\text{age (years)} + 16}{4}$$

PERFORMING CARDIOPULMONARY RESUSCITATION (CPR)

I. Airway (most pediatric arrests are respiratory events)
   A. Determine unresponsiveness
   B. Activate emergency medical service
   C. Observe for obstruction, which is most common precipitating event in arrest
   D. Clear oropharynx of secretions and/or vomitus
   E. Open airway
      1. Tilt head/lift chin
      2. Thrust jaw
      3. Maintain cervical spine alignment: do not hyperextend neck
      4. Insert oral/nasal airway to prevent airway obstruction

II. Breathing
   A. Determine breathlessness (look, listen, feel for breathing for 3–5 sec)
   B. Ventilate using bag-valve mask until placement of ETT or mouth-to-mouth is used in the field
   C. Give 2 slow rescue breaths with force sufficient to raise chest
   D. If airway obstructed, reposition and reattempt rescue breaths
      1. 5 abdominal thrusts (children >1 yr old)
      2. 5 back blows (children <1 yr old)
      3. 5 chest thrusts (children <1 yr old)
      4. Tongue-jaw lift and finger sweep in children >8 yr (in children <8 yr, finger sweep only if foreign object is visible)
   E. Rescue breathing only (pulse present)
      1. Children <8 yr old: 1 breath q 3 sec (approximately 20 per min)
      2. Children >8 yr old: 1 breath q 5 sec (approximately 12 per min)

III. Circulation
   A. Palpate pulse after rescue breaths
      1. Carotid in children >1 yr old
      2. Brachial in children <1 yr old
   B. If pulse is absent, begin chest compressions (need firm surface)
      1. Find chest landmarks
         a. Child >1 yr old: lower sternum, 2 fingerbreaths above sternal notch
         b. Child <1 yr old: 1 fingerbreath below intersection of sternum and imaginary line between nipples
      2. Compression rate
         a. Children <1 yr old: 100–120 per min
         b. Children 1–8 yr old: 100 per min
         c. Children >8 yr old: 80–100 per min
      3. Compression-breath ratio
         a. Children <1 yr old: 1 breath; 5 compressions
         b. Children >1 yr old: 2 breaths; 15 compressions
      4. Compression depth
         a. Children <1 yr old: 1/2–1 inch
         b. Children 1–8 yr old: 1–1½ inches
         c. Children >8 yr old: 1½–2 inches

Recent studies have documented the benefits of caregiver presence during CPR. The Emergency Nurses Association supports the option of family presence during resuscitation efforts. Be familiar with your institution's policies and procedures on caregiver presence during resuscitation.

INFECTION CONTROL

Standard precautions for infection control are designed to reduce the risk of transmission of bloodborne and other pathogens. There are five main routes of transmission: contact, droplet, airborne, common vehicle, and vector-borne. Standard precaution guidelines are designed to interrupt the mode of transmission. Standard precautions involve the use of barrier protection, such as gloves, goggles, gown, and masks, to prevent contamination from blood, all body fluids, secretions and excretions (except sweat), nonintact skin, and mucous membranes. Standard precautions are designed for *all* clients to reduce the risk of transmission for both recognized and unrecognized infection sources.

The following basic principles should be observed:

- Wash hands between clients and after contact with blood, body fluids, secretions, and excretions and after contact with articles or equipment contaminated by them.
- Wash hands immediately after removal of gloves.
- Wear gloves when touching blood, body fluids, secretions, excretions, nonintact skin, mucous membranes, or contaminated articles.
- Remove gloves and wash hands between client care.
- If client-care activities can generate splashes or sprays of blood or body fluids, wear masks, eye protection, or face shields.
- Wear a gown if soiling of clothes from blood or body fluids is likely.
- Wash hands after removal of gown.
- Clean equipment between client use and discard single-use items.
- Keep contaminated linens in leak-proof bags and handle in a manner to prevent skin and mucous-membrane exposure.
- Discard sharp instruments and needles in a puncture-resistant container. The Centers for Disease Control and Prevention (CDC) recommends that needles be uncapped for disposal or capped by use of a mechanical device.
- Determine reason for isolation and mode of transmission.

Isolation Category

- *Airborne precautions* apply to clients with known or suspected infections transmittable by the airborne route (e.g., measles, varicella, tuberculosis [TB]); special air handling and ventilation required; client must be in private room; mask or respiratory protection device is necessary
- *Droplet precautions* apply to clients with known or suspected infections transmittable by the droplet route (e.g., *H. influenzae* infections [meningitis, pneumonia, epiglottitis, sepsis, diphtheria, mycoplasm

pneumonia, pertussis, scarlet fever, rubella]); droplets are generated during sneezing, coughing, and talking; special air handling and ventilation are not required; place in private room or with cohort clients; masks are necessary

- *Contact precautions* are used to reduce the risk of transmission by direct or indirect contact; apply to clients with GI, respiratory, skin/wound infections, RSV; place in private room or with cohort clients; gloves, gowns, and masks (if spraying possible) are necessary

Isolation for TB

- TB isolation practices should be used in all clients with known or suspected TB.
- Client should be placed in a negative airflow private room with door closed.
- Health care workers must use a high-efficiency particulate air (HEPA) respirator or an N95 particulate respirator mask when entering the room. Check institution policies for type of mask available, reusability, storage, and proper fitting requirements.

CLINICAL SKILLS AND TIPS

To Encourage Fluid Intake

Melt popsicles in microwave until slushy. Child can then eat it with a spoon or straw. Feels good on sore throats. Offer a 5- to 10-cc syringe. Show child how to draw up liquid and squirt it in his or her mouth. Works best with 3–10 yr olds. Improves intake because it is fun. Can also give child a small medicine cup to drink from.

To Encourage Deep Breathing

Have child blow bubbles or a pinwheel. Can have child "blow out the light" with a pen light. Have child blow a cotton ball across the bedside table into a paper cup and pretend it is a soccer or hockey goal.

To Decrease Gagging

Gently press back on the chin to help stop gag reflex. Works best in young infants.

To Calm Fussy Babies

If you have ensured baby is not hungry nor needs changing, check to be sure IV has not infiltrated. This is the most common cause of inconsolable fussy babies. Expose IV as much as necessary to ensure patency. Compare extremities for size and shape to determine swelling. If IV is patent, try rocking motions, soothing voice, singing, or playing music to calm baby.

To Start IV in Infants

Best site for young infants is the head. It causes less restriction in movement and the least amount of disturbance in achievement of developmental tasks. Infants forget it is there and leave it alone. If it infiltrates, there is little tissue damage because circulation to area is less impaired than in the extremities. When the scalp is used, save a lock of the infant's hair that is shaved for the caregiver to put in the baby book to remember first "hair cut." This helps ease caregiver's chagrin over infant having his or her head shaved.

Warm Soaks

Warm soaks to extremities stay warm longer if extremity is wrapped in a warm wash cloth and then "diapered" with a disposable diaper. The plastic helps keep warmth in longer and keeps bed from getting wet.

SPECIMEN COLLECTION TIPS

Urine Collection

Infants

Clean area and allow to dry. Prepare area with Benzoin if skin is intact, let dry until sticky and attach pediatric urine bag. Can extract urine from bag with small-gauge needle and leave bag attached if more urine is needed. Young infants have a reflex that, if they are suspended supine on the nurse's hand, he or she can press at base of spine and gently stroke upward with two fingers. This causes infant to arch back, raise buttocks in the air, cry, and void if bladder is full. Allows for quick collection of specimen in bag or cup held under infant.

Toddlers/Preschoolers

Place hat-type specimen collection container in the hole in child's potty chair. Then child can void normally and not have to "perform" by voiding in a cup.

School-Aged Children/Adolescents

Easier to collect clean-catch specimen if he or she sits backward on toilet. This makes child spread his or her legs for cleaning and to hold the cup.

Stool Collection

If you need to collect loose stool in infants to send for electrolytes, can bag the anus using a pediatric urine bag. May want to put plastic wrap in diaper to use to scrape stool for collection.

Blood Collection

Warm extremity before capillary draws. Wipe area with alcohol again after the stick to increase blood flow. Squeezing extremity or digit can increase hemolysis and artificially elevate potassium results. Capillary hematocrit (Hct) can be 5%–10% higher than venous Hct. For venous collections, antecubital vein is best for all age groups and hurts less than using veins on hand or foot.

CHAPTER 6

COMMON HEALTH PROBLEMS

ACUTE GLOMERULONEPHRITIS (AGN)

Brief Description

AGN is a disorder in which immune complexes deposit along the glomerular membrane. Most cases follow streptococcal, pneumococcal, or viral infections. Glomerular capillary loops become swollen and infiltrated, causing decreased filtration of plasma. This noninfectious renal disorder primarily affects school-aged children. Recovery is spontaneous and children generally recover completely.

History and Physical Assessment Findings

Urine is smoke colored, tea colored, or grossly bloody. Proteinuria is present. Patients commonly report history of strep throat or other infection 2 wk before symptoms. Urine output decreased. Child has edema (especially facial and periorbital). Physical examination findings (e.g., edema, increased blood pressure [BP], increased weight) vary depending on level of renal involvement. Edematous phase can last up to 3 wk with child feeling apathetic during that time. Increasing urine output and decreasing weight indicate improvement.

Nursing Care

Supportive nursing care indicated. Children with mild cases (normal BP and urine output) treated as outpatients. Close assessment of vital signs, weight, and intake and output essential. Child may be placed on fluid and sodium restrictions if urine output significantly low. Antihypertensive medications may be indicated. Antibiotics are prescribed if child has persistent streptococcal infection.

Related Nursing Diagnoses

- Fluid volume excess
- Risk for injury

- Potential body-image disturbance
- Fatigue

AGGRESSIVENESS

Brief Description

Children with aggressiveness exhibit behavior in which they attempt to hurt another person or destroy another's property. Often the behavior is unprovoked and is exhibited through physical attacks, destruction of property, extreme impulsivity, and noncompliance. Frustration, modeling another's behavior, and reinforcement seem to increase aggressive behavior. This behavioral problem is influenced by biologic, sociocultural, and familial variables.

History and Physical Assessment Findings

History of hostility, combativeness, and fighting common. Majority have associated social impairments, psychiatric disorders, or adult criminal behavior.

Nursing Care

Treatment includes caregiver management training, teaching child new coping skills, family therapy, and psychopharmacologic intervention. Early intervention is the goal. Referral to psychiatrist or psychologist is often necessary.

Related Nursing Diagnoses

- Risk for injury
- Social isolation
- Impaired social interaction
- Interrupted family processes
- Risk for violence, directed at others
- Ineffective individual coping

ANXIETY

Brief Description

Children with anxiety have general uneasiness and apprehension. Anxiety is different from fear; fears are more specific in nature and generally are limited problems that disappear with growth. Anxiety usually manifests as panic attack. Panic attacks are unexpected events.

History and Physical Assessment Findings

Panic attacks are associated with at least four of the following symptoms: shortness of breath (SOB), dizziness/faintness, palpitations or tachycardia, shakiness, sweating, feeling of choking, nausea/abdominal discomfort, numbness/tingling, flushing, chest pain/discomfort, fear of dying, and fear of losing control.

Nursing Care

Therapy with mental health professional indicated for children with anxiety. Psychopharmacologic treatment has not proven effective in children with anxiety disorders.

Related Nursing Diagnoses

- Death anxiety
- Ineffective individual coping
- Sleep pattern disturbance

ASTHMA (REACTIVE AIRWAY DISEASE)

Brief Description

Asthma is a chronic pulmonary disease that results from a wide range of stimuli (e.g., pollen, dust, viruses, smoke, strong odors, roach dander, animals). Results in increased irritability of tracheobronchial tree with airway obstruction of varying degrees. Asthma episode may or may not be reversible following therapy or spontaneously. Children are more vulnerable to airway obstruction because of their small airway and compromised collateral ventilation. Narrowing of airway caused by smooth muscle contraction of airway (bronchospasm), edema and inflammation of tracheobronchial mucosa, and excessive secretion of submucosal glands, which causes mucous plugging.

Classification of Asthma Severity

Step 1: Mild Intermittent Asthma

Symptoms ≤2x/wk
Asymptomatic with normal peak expiratory flow (PEF) between exacerbations
Exacerbations brief (from few hours to few days) with varying intensity
Nighttime symptoms ≤2x/mo
Forced expiratory volume over 1 min (FEV_1)/PEF ≥80% of predicted value, with variability <20%

Step 2: Mild Persistent Asthma

Symptoms >2x/wk but <1x/day
Exacerbations may affect activity
Nighttime symptoms >2x/wk
FEV_1/PEF 80% of predicted value with variability of 20%–30%

Step 3: Moderate Persistent Asthma

Daily symptoms
Daily use of inhaled, short-acting β_2-agonist
Exacerbations affect activity
Exacerbations $\geq$2x/wk; may last for days
Nighttime symptoms >1x/wk
FEV_1/PEF between 60% and 80% of predicted value with 30% variability

Step 4: Severe Persistent Asthma

Continual symptoms
Limited physical activity
Frequent exacerbations
Frequent nighttime symptoms
FEV_1/PEF <60% of predicted value with >30% variability (Kemper, 1997)

Diagnostic Tests

The following tests need to be performed:

- Complete blood cell count (CBC)—leukocytosis occasionally found, eosinophilia frequently found
- Serum immunoglobulin E (IgE)
- Pulmonary function tests
- PEF
- Chest X ray
- Allergy testing

History and Physical Assessment Findings

Obtain thorough history including medications routinely used at home. Children with asthma often have history of eczema, recurrent bronchitis, and persistent cough. Symptoms usually worse at night. Assess exposure to triggers, especially environmental tobacco smoke (ETS). Respiratory assessment should include respiratory rate, presence of dyspnea, retractions, nasal flaring, and use of accessory muscles. Skin color and capillary refill time should be noted. Lungs should be auscultated for unequal breath sounds, crackles, and/or wheezes. Cardiac rate and rhythm should be assessed, especially during drug therapy.

Nursing Care

Assess child's and caregiver's understanding of disease process and use of medications to manage. Provide client teaching related to avoidance of allergens and/or triggers. Administer drug therapy and teach caregivers and child what drugs do to help asthma and whether they are short- or long-term use drugs. Short-acting β_2-agonists such as albuterol may be used PO or by inhalation. Cromolyn and inhaled steroids are long-acting, preventive drugs. Steroids are also given PO or IV for acute exacerbations. Provide oxygen p.r.n. and monitor pulse oximeter readings. Place in Fowler's or semi-Fowler's position to facilitate breathing. Provide teaching related to home care including use of PEF meter and how to manage asthma according to PEF reading. Children >6 yr can be taught to use PEF meter; all children discharged with diagnosis of asthma should have written management plan that is reviewed with caregiver and child and a copy sent home with them.

Related Nursing Diagnoses

- Ineffective breathing patterns
- Ineffective airway clearance
- Ineffective health maintenance

ATTENTION DEFICIT HYPERACTIVITY DISORDER (ADHD)

Brief Description

ADHD is a chronic neurobehavioral disorder that can interfere with a child's ability to inhibit behavior, function effectively in goal-oriented activities, and/or regulate activity level in developmentally appropriate ways. Three behavioral subtypes are defined by the American Psychiatric Association *Diagnostic and Statistical Manual of Mental Disorders, 4th Edition* (DSM-IV). Subtypes are predominately inattentive, predominately hyperactive/impulsive, and combined. Symptoms usually start after child is 7 years old and can be diagnosed after they have persisted ≥6 mo. Some children can be diagnosed earlier, but rarely before age 4 years for accurate diagnosis. Underlying problem is still unclear; however, there are many theories. One is that affected child cannot produce enough norepinephrine, a neurochemical transmitter, to allow messages to be transmitted effectively from one neuron to another to complete the transmission.

History and Physical Assessment Findings

Disorder usually affects all aspects of child's life but is most pervasive in school-related activities. No specific diagnostic measures are currently available. Diagnosis based on evaluation of child's behavior in multiple settings, such as school, home, and day care, by multiple people having contact with child. A plethora of behavioral checklists is available to aid caregivers, teachers, and school nurses in assessing behavioral characteristics. Initial assessment should include questions about chronic problems, behavioral problems, how child is managed at home (e.g., behavior modification), routines, and medications and times of administration. Also assess when medication seems to be wearing off and how long it lasts in current setting. Ritalin (usually first drug used) lasts 3–5 hr.

Nursing Care

Provide safe environment, try as much as possible to maintain routines as they are at home, and ensure provision of medication at a time most appropriate for child's care. Communicate to family and all caregivers that child has a behavior problem that has multiple origins including an underlying central nervous system (CNS) basis and needs understanding, reassurance, and routine in a new setting. Encourage family involvement in plan and care.

Related Nursing Diagnoses

- Potential for self-esteem disturbance
- Impaired social interaction
- Interrupted family processes
- Risk for impaired parenting

AUTISM

Brief Description

Autism is a complex developmental syndrome involving impaired brain functioning, intellectual deficits, and behavioral deficits. Children with autism demonstrate bizarre social interactions, communication, and behavior. Generally manifests in children ages 18–36 mo. More commonly found in males. Autism is usually severely disabling.

History and Physical Assessment Findings

Abnormal electroencephalogram (EEG), seizures, delayed development of hand dominance, persistent primitive reflexes, elevated blood serotonin, and cerebellar vermal hypoplasia. Classic sign is inability to maintain eye contact with another person. Majority have some degree of mental retardation.

Nursing Care

Most children require lifelong adult supervision. No cure for this syndrome exists. Children with autism need highly structured and intensive behavioral modification programs; these have shown to be most effective therapy. Goal of care is to promote positive reinforcement, increase social awareness, develop communication skills, and decrease unacceptable behaviors. Providing structured environment is critical aspect of care. During child's hospitalization, caregivers are essential to care planning and should remain with child as much as possible. Physical contact should be avoided because it is distressing to children with autism.

Related Nursing Diagnoses

- Impaired social interaction
- Impaired verbal communication
- Risk for caregiver role strain
- Disturbed thought processes
- Delayed growth and development
- Risk for self-mutilation
- Risk for injury

BRONCHIOLITIS

Brief Description

Bronchiolitis is an acute viral infection of the small airways in the lower respiratory tract causing airway hypersensitivity, edema, and inflammation. Majority of cases result from respiratory syncytial virus (RSV). Rate of infection peaks in months between November and March; average age of those affected is 2–9 mo. Bronchiolitis is one of the most common causes of pediatric hospitalization, although most children with this illness are managed at home. This infection may be life-threatening especially in children with cardiac and respiratory disease history (e.g., congenital heart disease, bronchopulmonary dysplasia).

History and Physical Assessment Findings

Usually a history of recent upper respiratory infection with symptoms of cough, nasal stuffiness, and fever. As illness progresses, symptoms become more severe and result in increased work of breathing. Usually an increased respiratory rate, shallow respiratory pattern, nasal flaring, retractions, and tachycardia. Children with severe illness may exhibit decreased air entry and lethargy. Diagnosis made on basis of the history, physical examination, chest X ray (shows hyperinflation/inflammation), and positive viral culture (nasopharyngeal wash).

Nursing Care

Ongoing close assessment necessary. Because of structure of child's airway, deteriorating changes can occur very rapidly. Treatment generally supportive in nature. Oxygen and respiratory therapies often ordered. O_2 mist tent may be used. Continuous pulse oximetry indicated, especially early in illness. Interventions aimed at keeping airway clear should be implemented (e.g., suctioning, increasing height of head of bed). Nebulized bronchodilators (e.g., albuterol) often ordered. Use of ribavirin (via small-particle aerosol) usually reserved for those with severe symptoms and those with preexisting cardiopulmonary states. Because of teratogenic effects of ribavirin, pregnant health care workers should not provide care for children receiving ribavirin therapy.

Related Nursing Diagnoses

- Ineffective breathing pattern
- Ineffective tissue perfusion
- Risk for deficient fluid volume
- Fear
- Anxiety
- Deficient knowledge

CANCER

Brief Description

Cause of cancer in children is unknown, but genetic alterations resulting in unregulated proliferation of cells, genetic inheritance, chromosomal abnormalities, immune system suppression, Epstein-Barr virus, environmental agents, power line exposure, and certain drugs all have been proposed as possible causative factors in various types of cancers in children.

Presenting Signs and Symptoms

Fever
Pain
Limping
Anemia
Bruising or petechiae
Infection
Fatigue
Painless abdominal mass
Weight loss
Palpable lymph nodes
Behavioral changes
Night sweats
Seizure activity
Neurologic changes

Leukocoria (white reflection in pupil)
Early morning headaches

Diagnostic Work-up

History and physical examination
Laboratory studies
Bone marrow aspiration
Diagnostic imaging
Surgical staging, biopsy

Treatment Modalities

Child usually placed on a protocol involving any or all of the following:
Surgery
Chemotherapy
Radiation
Bone marrow transplant

Common Types of Cancer in Children

Leukemia

Leukemia is a group of malignant disorders of the bone marrow and lymphatic system and is the most common form of childhood cancer. Two forms recognized in children are *acute lymphoid leukemia* (ALL), which is the most common, and *acute myelogenous leukemia* (AML).

Lymphoma

Lymphoma is a group of neoplastic diseases that arise from the lymphoid and hemopoietic systems and are divided into Hodgkin's and non-Hodgkin's lymphoma (NHL). Both have four stages depending on tumor spread and lymph node involvement.

Brain Tumors

Brain tumors are the most common solid tumors in children and include the following types:

- Low- or high-grade astrocytoma—Most common pediatric brain tumor that infiltrates the brain parenchyma without distinct boundaries
- Medulloblastoma (primitive neuroectodermal tumor [PNET])—Fast growing, highly malignant
- Cerebellar astrocytoma—Slow growing if low grade
- Brainstem glioma—Often grows very large before causes symptoms; most are highly resistant to therapy

Ependymoma—Most invade the ventricles, obstructing cerebrospinal
id (CSF) flow

stoma

na, tumors arise from embryonic neural crest cells, so major-
ne from the adrenal gland or from the retroperitoneal sym-
ost common primary site is the abdomen. Also has staging
umor dissemination.

umors

are two types of *bone tumors:*

- Osteogenic sarcoma—Most common type of bone tumor in children that arises from the osseous tissue. More than half occur in the femur, especially the distal part, with the rest involving the humerus, tibia, pelvis, jaw, and phalanges.
- Ewing's sarcoma (PNET of the bone)-—Aises in the marrow spaces of the bone.

Other Solid Tumors

- Wilms' tumor (nephroblastoma)—Tumor of the kidney; has hereditary component. Most common intraabdominal tumor of children.
- Rhabdomyosarcoma—Most common soft tissue tumor in children; arises in striated muscle. Most common sites are head and neck, especially the orbit.
- Retinoblastoma—Malignant tumor; arises from retina. Can be inherited.

Side Effects of Treatment

Infection
Hemorrhage
Anemia
Altered nutrition
Neurologic problems
Hemorrhagic cystitis
Alopecia
Nausea and vomiting
Mucosal ulceration
Lowered body defenses

Nursing Care

Prepare client and family for diagnostic and treatment procedures. Involve play therapy as appropriate. Provide support for family during diagnostic and treatment processes by answering questions; encouraging verbalization of fears and concerns; and involving social services, chaplains, and support groups as appropriate. Administer chemotherapy as ordered and monitor for side effects of all medications. Protect from infection and administer antiemetics before and p.r.n. after chemotherapy to prevent and treat nausea and vomiting. Assess for pain and administer analgesics as ordered; implement pain management techniques. Ensure adequate nutrition by encouraging intake of small portions of anything tolerated by the child. Provide meticulous skin care, including oral mucous membranes, to help prevent breakdown. Encourage developmentally appropriate activities. Provide education about disease process and needed care as well as for home care as appropriate.

Related Nursing Diagnoses

- Risk for injury
- Risk for infection
- Risk for deficient fluid volume
- Impaired oral mucous membranes
- Imbalanced nutrition: less than body requirements
- Impaired skin integrity
- Disturbed body image
- Pain
- Fear
- Interrupted family processes
- Ineffective health maintenance
- Anticipatory grieving
- Deficient knowledge
- Deficient diversional activity

CARE OF THE CHILD AND FAMILY WITH CHRONIC ILLNESS

The number of children with chronic diseases and conditions are increasing. These children and their families have unique responses, needs, and nursing care requirements.

Effect on Child

The impact of chronic illness on a child is influenced by age of onset. Unpredictability can lead to frequent hospitalizations and appointments with health care practitioners that interrupt normalcy. May have associated pain and discomfort. Child may have misinformation or not enough information and fear the unknown. Growth and development may be restricted, which makes these children different from their peers. They may be unable to participate in normal activities, which also makes them feel different from their peers. May have decreased feelings of worth and feel guilty for daily care requirements.

Child's Response

Child may respond by being angry, uncooperative, and belligerent. May show signs of depression, resignation, or confusion. May also feel isolated and withdrawn, although some children seem to rise to each new challenge and adapt quite well.

Effect on Family

Grieve for loss of normal child and his or her potential. Feel a strain on all relationships, stress over daily care requirements and financial burden, loss of control, and isolation.

Caregiver's Response

Type of chronic illness and amount of positive feedback from child affect caregiver's response. Caregivers may go through denial, grief, guilt, anger, helplessness, fear, and loneliness. These feelings may potentiate at every missed milestone, such as first steps, first day at school, or getting a driver's license.

Sibling's Response

May feel forgotten and less important than and jealous of sick sibling. May get angry and resent caregivers being away all the time. May feel guilty, sad, isolated, or lonely, and may act out to get attention.

Nursing Intervention

General

Use primary nurse as much as possible and admit to same unit in hospital each admission. Use developmental approach instead of one based on age to help emphasize abilities and not disabilities. Focus on strengths. Encourage normalcy as much as is realistic. As families learn about their child and his or her condition, they become experts for that child and need to be recognized as such.

Child

Depends on developmental level and condition. Assess child's understanding of illness and how he or she is responding and adapting. Provide support for coping and allow and encourage expression of feelings. Promote normal growth and development. Prepare for changes and treatments. Encourage participation in and responsibility for care and control as much as possible. Encourage peer and sibling support and help with care; help them understand expectations and responsibilities. Focus on abilities. Encourage association with peers with same problems if possible, and encourage involvement in decision making.

Caregivers

Assess how well caregivers are adapting to child's illness. Determine and provide knowledge, skills, and resources needed to help them adapt. Provide information on normal growth and development so they can encourage development of their child. Encourage involvement of all caregivers. Clarify needs of each caregiver; they may be in different stages of adapting because of different amounts of contact with child and health care system. Encourage normalization and realistic expectations of child and of family functioning. Encourage open communication. Allow verbalization of frustrations and feelings, and respond in a caring, nonjudgmental, nondefensive manner. Help caregivers get involved in support groups if appropriate and help them set up their own support systems.

Siblings

Encourage visitation and involvement in care during hospitalization if appropriate for sibling's age and child's condition. Assess sibling's understanding of child's illness and his or her adjustment to it. Provide supportive communication. Encourage phone calls to caregivers and sick child. Give positive strokes when present and recognize sibling's presence and feelings.

CARING FOR THE DYING CHILD AND THE FAMILY

Death is a difficult nursing situation because it causes nurses to examine their feelings about death—their own and others. Working with dying children and their families can be both challenging and rewarding. To be most effective, nurses need to be aware of how different age groups conceptualize and react to death—their own and others.

Perceptions by Age Groups

Infants/Toddlers

Concept: None

Reaction to own impending: Take cues from loved ones' responses

Reaction to death of others: React to the separation and loss of consistency by regressing, becoming irritable, and developing sleeping and eating problems.

Preschoolers (3–5 years)

Concept: Is separation; temporary, gradual, and reversible

Reaction to own impending: Is punishment for bad thoughts or actions

Reaction to death of others: May feel guilty, as if their thoughts or actions were responsible; may regress or show denial with inappropriate behavior

School-aged Children (6–11 years)

Concept: Is not reversible but also is not inevitable; may see it as destructive or look for natural or physical explanations

Reaction to own impending: May show fear of the unknown; need help to maintain control of own body. May be verbally uncooperative because of fear; show "flight or fight" reaction

Reaction to death of others: Feel guilt and responsibility; ask many questions to help arrange facts into concrete and logical understanding

Adolescents (12–18 years)

Concept: Is irreversible, universal, and inevitable. Is a personal but far-off event. Explain it physiologically and theologically.

Reaction to own impending: Reject death because it interferes with their establishment of identity. Become alienated from their peers and unable to talk to caregivers. Use denial and rationalization. Are present oriented and worry about physical changes that may further alienate them from their peers.

Reaction to death of others: Feel guilt and shame. This group has more difficulty coping with death than do the other age groups and may be unable to accept support.

Caregiver Responses

Initial (When informed of life-threatening illness or condition of child)

Shock, disbelief
Anger
Overprotectiveness
Anxiety
Ambivalence

After the Loss

Shock, confusion, decreased sense of reality
Guilt, anger
Sorrow
Depression
Loneliness, yearning
Helplessness, despair, fear
Reorganization, reconciliation, relief

Caregivers may be in different stages of acceptance and may respond differently. Caregivers may have reached acceptance before nurse does. May be reconciled to death of child long before child dies. Child's death after lengthy, painful illness may be a relief. Need to be helped to understand that this is alright and should not feel guilty for their feelings.

Sibling Responses

Siblings respond according to their age group and developmental stage. Reaction also depends on caregivers' reactions, amount of time they have had to adjust, and amount of involvement and inclusion they have had. Often feel isolated and guilty. May also feel that they are not as important as child who died and that they need to replace that child and be strong, be good, and not talk about their sibling. May have been sheltered and left out.

Nursing Care

Nurses may need help dealing with their own feelings before they are able to help the dying child and his or her family. Seek assistance from experienced nurses, social worker, or chaplain. All nurses are initially uncomfortable because it forces us face our children's and our own mortality. Be careful to not impose your own views, values, or explanations on the family.

Child

The dying child needs accurate, honest information and time to think it out. Process needs to be gradual with increasingly open communication between child, caregivers, and nurse. When child asks questions, ask what he or she thinks is happening to find out what he or she understands, how he or she feels, and what child really wants to know. Be sure to discuss with caregivers before about how they want to handle communication and what they want child to know. Even though open communication is best, it is still the caregivers' right to determine what they feel is best for the child. Help correct any misinformation.

Family

Assess resources and ability to cope; intervene and refer as necessary. Caregivers also need honest and complete information to empower them to make appropriate choices. They need information on how to tell the child, siblings, and other family members. They need an opportunity to express their feelings in a supportive environment. Respect their wishes in regard to what they want child to know, but help them realize that trust fosters trust. After the death of the child, stay with the family or have a chaplain or social worker available. Ensure the child's dignity. Encourage expression of memories and feelings. Answer questions honestly. Allow them to stay with the child as long as they wish. Give them time and privacy to say goodbye. Help with arrangements, ensure closure, encourage current ties with nursing staff.

CENTRAL NERVOUS SYSTEM INFECTIONS

Brief Description

CNS infections include bacterial meningitis, aseptic/viral meningitis, encephalitis, and brain abscess. Both bacterial and viral meningitis result in inflammation of the meninges. Bacterial meningitis is more serious than viral meningitis and is sometimes fatal. Encephalitis is inflammation of the brain; often the meninges are also inflamed. Common pathogens associated with bacterial meningitis include *Haemophilus influenzae, Streptococcus pneumoniae, Neisseria meningitides,* group B streptococcus, *Staphylococcus aureus,* and pseudomonas. Aseptic meningitis is most commonly caused by enterovirus. Encephalitis usually follows other infections such as measles, varicella, mumps, herpes, Epstein-Barr infection, and influenza. Common pathogens associated with brain abscesses include *S. aureus,* group A streptococcus, *H. influenza,* gram-negative enteric bacteria, and fungi.

History and Physical Assessment Findings

Children with CNS infections may have history of immune compromise, travel outside of country, lack of immunization, and vector exposure (e.g., mosquito). Generally exhibit signs and symptoms such as nuchal rigidity, headache, behavior changes, seizures, photophobia, cranial nerve alterations, and fever. Positive Kernig's or Brudzinski sign may be present. Depending on the causative factor, children may also exhibit other signs such as rash (petechiae/purpura), vomiting, and diarrhea. CSF examination yields organisms and alterations in cell count, protein, and glucose. Blood and urine cultures may also be positive. CBC results demonstrate increase in white blood cells (WBCs).

Nursing Care

Initial care is considered an emergency. Careful assessment of neurologic status required. Child is placed in isolation, and standard precautions and droplet precautions are used until pathogen is identified. First priority of care for children with bacterial CNS infections is to administer IV antibiotics. Doses may be required for up to 3 wk depending on organism and virulence. Corticosteroids (e.g., dexamethasone), anticonvulsants, and antipyretics often given. Important to administer steroids before or with first dose of antibiotics. Antiviral (e.g., acyclovir) may be prescribed for those with aseptic meningitis. Surgery or aspiration may be indicated in children with brain abscesses. Accurate measurement of intake and output necessary; child may be placed on fluid restriction to prevent cerebral edema, increased intracranial pressure (IP), and syndrome of inappropriate antidiuretic hormone secretion (SIADH). Reduction of environmental stimuli recommended.

Related Nursing Diagnoses

- Infection
- Hyperthermia
- Ineffective tissue perfusion
- Pain
- Impaired social interaction
- Disturbed sensory perception
- Risk for ineffective family coping

COMMUNICABLE DISEASES

Chickenpox (Varicella)

Infective Organism. Varicella-zoster virus (VZV) is a herpesvirus.

Sources. Humans

Transmission. Direct contact with respiratory secretions; also airborne

Incubation Period. Usually 14–16 days

Signs and Symptoms. Pruritic rash begins on trunk as macules and progresses to vesicles and crusting. Child may have slight fever and decreased appetite.

Isolation. Airborne and contact precautions for ≥5 days after rash begins and for as long as rash is vesicular. For exposed susceptible clients, airborne and contact precautions for days 8–21 after onset in index client.

Nursing Care. Symptomatic. No aspirin because of increased risk of Reye's syndrome. Acetaminophen may delay crusting but can be used to control fever. Tepid bath with cornstarch may help with itching. Administer diphenhydramine hydrochloride (Benadryl) or hydroxyzine hydrochloride (Atarax) as ordered for itching. Keep child's nails short. Teach older child to push on itching lesions instead of scratching. Keep child cool to decrease itching and lesion formation. Sometimes treated with IV or PO acyclovir (IV for immunocompromised patients), but not recommended routinely for uncomplicated varicella in otherwise healthy child.

Complications. Local cellulitis from secondary infections, encephalitis, and Reye's syndrome.

Human Immunodeficiency Virus (HIV) Infection

Infective Organism. Human immunodeficiency virus type 1

Sources. Humans

Transmission. Predominant modes are via exposure to blood, semen, cervical secretions, and human milk from sexual contact; percutaneous or mucous membrane exposure, vertical from mother to infant at or around time of birth; and breastfeeding.

Incubation Period. Variable from months to years. Perinatally infected median age of onset is age 3 years. Those who acquire HIV other than perinatally usually develop serum antibodies to HIV within 6–12 wk after infection.

Signs and Symptoms. Can present in any system. Most common manifestations include generalized lymphadenopathy, hepatomegaly and splenomegaly, failure to thrive, recurrent or persistent oral candidiasis, recurrent diarrhea, parotitis, cardiomyopathy, hepatitis, nephropathy, and/or CNS disease. Also may show developmental delay, lymphoid interstitial pneumonitis (LIP), recurrent invasive bacterial infections, and opportunistic infections such as *Pneumocystis carinii* pneumonia (PCP).

Diagnostic Testing.

- HIV enzyme-linked immunosorbent assay (ELISA)—Screening test for HIV antibody.
- HIV western blot—Confirmatory test used to check validity of ELISA test because western blot more precisely detects presence of antibodies to specific antigens.

The aforementioned tests are accurate in children >18 mo.

- HIV p24 antigen assay—Tests for protein that surrounds the ribonucleic acid (RNA) and for reverse transcriptase of HIV
- HIV deoxyribonucleic acid (DNA) polymerase chain reaction (PCR)—Standard current diagnostic test
- HIV culture—HIV culture and HIV PCR are the most sensitive and specific tests to determine HIV infection in children who were perinatally exposed

Classification. As of 1994 (Centers for Disease Control and Prevention [CDC], 1994), children with HIV infection are classified by three immunologic and three clinical categories.

Immunologic categories categorize by severity of immunosuppression caused by HIV infection. Age-specific CD4 counts and T-lymphocyte percentages determine category.

1. No evidence of suppression
2. Evidence of moderate suppression
3. Severe suppression

Clinical categories are used to provide a staging classification.

N. Not symptomatic
A. Mildly symptomatic
B. Moderately symptomatic
C. Severely symptomatic

The best prognosis is for a child classified as N1; poorest is C3. The CDC has established specific parameters and definitions. An E prefix means perinatally exposed.

Isolation. Universal blood and body fluid precautions

Nursing Care. Depends somewhat on child's classification and condition. Many have multiple hospitalizations and need same care as other children with chronic or life-threatening illnesses. Need to help support family and child emotionally by listening and helping set up services as needed. Use social services and all resources available in the community. Growth and development surveillance important. Protect from secondary infections with good handwashing and protective isolation as warranted by CD4 and T-lymphocyte counts. Help keep hydrated, maintain good nutrition, and encourage development as much as tolerated. Administer antibiotics and antifungals as ordered. Provide education about transmission and prevention of HIV infection.

Complications. Failure to thrive or HIV wasting syndrome, loss of developmental milestones, multiple and persistent infections, LIP, PCP, HIV encephalopathy, and death.

Kawasaki Disease

Infective Organism. Unknown. Epidemiologic and clinical features suggest infectious cause.

Sources. No evidence of human-to-human or common-source spread but incidence slightly higher in siblings of clients with this disease.

Incubation Period. Unknown

Signs and Symptoms. Disease occurs mostly in children <5 yr of age. Have fever for ≥5 days and at least four of the following five features, or fever and three of the features and evidence of coronary artery abnormalities. Features appear within several days of onset of fever and include the following: (1) injected bulbar conjunctiva without discharge; (2) red mouth and pharynx, strawberry tongue, and red, cracked lips; (3) generalized rash; (4) peeling and redness of palms and soles; and (5) unilateral cervical lymphadenopathy ≥1.5 cm in diameter.

Isolation. Standard precautions for hospitalized patients

Nursing Care. Supportive care. Administer anti-inflammatory therapy as ordered. Children usually receive high-dose immune globulin intravenous (IGIV) therapy and high-dose aspirin (80–100 mg/kg/24 hr q.i.d. and then decreased when fever is under control). Monitor aspirin levels, provide for comfort and nutrition, and be alert to signs and symptoms of congestive heart failure (CHF), murmurs, and arrhythmias.

Complications. Major complication is risk for development of coronary artery aneurysms.

Measles (Rubeola)

Infective Organism. RNA virus classified as morbillivirus

Sources. Humans

Transmission. Direct contact with droplets; less commonly airborne

Incubation Period. Usually 8–12 days

Signs and Symptoms. Fever, cough, coryza, conjunctivitis with photophobia, and Koplik's spots on posterior buccal mucosa, followed in 2–3 days by erythematous maculopapular rash beginning on face and spreading downward. Rash is confluent and turns a brownish color after 3–4 days. Skin may peel over heavily rashed areas.

Isolation. Airborne precautions for 4–5 days after onset of rash. Immunocompromised children need to be isolated for entire course of illness because of prolonged excretion of virus in respiratory secretions.

Nursing Care. Symptomatic. Bedrest, antipyretics, dim lights, cool mist vaporizer, tepid baths

Complications. Otitis media (OM), bronchopneumonia, croup, and diarrhea in young children; encephalitis; and rarely, subacute sclerosing panencephalitis (SSPE).

Mumps

Infective Organism. Paramyxovirus

Sources. Humans

Transmission. Direct contact via respiratory route

Incubation Period. Usually 16–18 days

Signs and Symptoms. Fever, headache, and malaise followed by swelling and pain of one or both parotid glands, although one-third of infections do not cause apparent salivary swelling

Isolation. Droplet precautions until 9 days after onset of parotid swelling

Nursing Care. Supportive. Bedrest, antipyretics, analgesics, increased fluids, soft bland diet, hot or cold compresses to parotid glands

Complications. Encephalitis (rare) or orchitis (more common in adults)

Pertussis (Whooping Cough)

Infective Organism. *Bordetella pertussis*

Sources. Humans

Transmission. Close contact via respiratory secretions

Incubation Period. 6–20 days, usually 7–10 days

Signs and Symptoms. Mild upper respiratory symptoms progressing to severe paroxysms of coughing with inspiratory "whoop" usually followed by vomiting. Fever, if present, is usually low grade. In infants <6 mo, apnea is common symptom and whoop often absent.

Isolation. Droplet precautions for 5 days after beginning effective therapy or until 3 wk after onset of cough if not treated with antimicrobial therapy

Nursing Care. Erythromycin usually drug of choice but others can be used. Administer drugs as ordered, otherwise supportive care with bedrest until no fever; encourage fluids and increase humidity via humidifier or tent. Refeed after vomiting. Observe for airway obstruction.

Complications. Pneumonia, seizures, hernia, prolapsed rectum, encephalopathy, and death

Disease is most severe in first year of life, especially for preterm infants.

Rotavirus

Infective Organism. Rotavirus, an RNA virus belonging to the family Reoviridae

Sources. Humans, mostly and possibly fomites

Transmission. Fecal-oral route. Found on toys and hard surfaces in day care centers. Also could have respiratory transmission.

Incubation Period. 1–3 days

Signs and Symptoms. Diarrhea usually preceded or accompanied by vomiting and low-grade fever.

Diagnostic Testing. Enzyme immunoassay (EIA) and latex agglutination assays for group A rotavirus-antigen detection in stool during diarrhea

Isolation. Strict contact precautions for duration of illness and hospitalization. Prolonged fecal shedding of low concentration of virus after recovery.

Nursing Care. Symptomatic. Prevent dehydration by administering IV fluids as ordered. Good skin care in diaper area. Educate caregiver about good handwashing technique and use of gloves with diaper changes.

Complications. Severe cases can cause dehydration with electrolyte imbalances; acidosis, which can lead to neurologic signs

Rubella (German Measles, Three-Day Measles)

Infective Organism. RNA virus classified as rubivirus

Sources. Humans

Transmission. Direct or droplet contact with nasal secretions. Some infants with congenital rubella shed virus in nasopharyngeal secretions and urine for $\geq$1 yr.

Incubation Period. 14–21 days, but usually 16–18 days

Signs and Symptoms. Postnatal: Pinkish-red maculopapular discrete rash beginning on face and progressing rapidly downward; covers body the first day. Disappears in order it came, usually by day 3. Accompanied in older children by low-grade fever and generalized lymphadenopathy, especially suboccipital, cervical, and postauricular. Transient polyarthralgia and polyarthritis common in adolescent girls.

Isolation. Postnatal: Droplet precautions for first 7 days after onset of rash. Congenital: Contact isolation; consider contagious until 1 yr old.

Nursing Care. Supportive. Antipyretics for fever and analgesics for discomfort

Complications. Encephalitis, thrombocytopenia (rare). Biggest complication is teratogenic effect on fetus.

Streptococcal Tonsillitis/Pharyngitis

Infective Organism. Group A β-hemolytic streptococci

Sources. Humans

Transmission. Contact with respiratory tract secretions

Incubation Period. Usually 2–5 days

Signs and Symptoms. Occurs at all ages but most commonly in school-aged children. Present with fever; sore throat; and swollen, tender tonsillar nodes, and can have palatal petechiae and white, strawberry tongue. Tonsils usually swollen and red and have yellow exudate. Toddlers present with moderate fever, serous rhinitis, irritability, and anorexia.

Isolation. Droplet precautions recommended until 24 hr after starting antibiotics.

Nursing Care. Obtain throat swab for rapid strep test or culture as ordered. Make sure to swab both tonsillar pillars and the posterior pharynx, taking care to avoid tongue by using tongue blade. Administer antibiotics as ordered. Provide for comfort measures and fever control p.r.n.

Tuberculosis (TB)

Infective Organism. *Mycobacterium tuberculosis*

Sources. Humans; children usually get it from infected adults

Transmission. Airborne inhalation from infected respiratory droplets from an adult or adolescent with infectious pulmonary tuberculosis

Incubation Period. From infection to TB skin test being positive is 2–12 wk. Risk for developing disease state is greatest in first 6 mo after infection and remains high for 2 yr. Most become dormant.

Signs and Symptoms. Positive Mantoux test using 5 tuberculin units of purified protein derivative (PPD) administered intradermally indicates infection. Tests should be read 48–72 hr after placement. Positivity interpreted as follows as recommended by the American Academy of Pediatrics

Committee on Infectious Diseases (American Academy of Pediatrics, 2000). These recommendations apply regardless of bacille Calmette-Guérin (BCG) vaccine administration.

Reaction ≥5 mm

- Children in close contact with persons with known or suspected infectious TB
- Children suspected to have TB because of positive chest X ray or clinical evidence of TB
- Children with immunosuppressive conditions including immunosuppressive dose of corticosteroids or HIV infection

Reaction ≥10 mm

- Children at increased risk of acquiring TB as a result of the following:
  - Young age (<4 yr old)
  - Medical risk factors of Hodgkin's lymphoma, diabetes mellitus, chronic renal failure, malnutrition
- Children with increased environmental exposure:
  - Foreign-born children or children of parents born in regions of increased TB incidence
  - Travel or exposure to high-prevalence regions of the world
- Frequent exposure to adults who are HIV infected; homeless; drug users; or residents of nursing homes, institutions, or prisons or migrant farm workers

Reaction ≥15 mm

- Children ≥4 yr old without any risk factors

Most children are asymptomatic. Early manifestations include lymphadenopathy, pulmonary involvement with or without consolidation, pleural effusion, miliary TB, and TB meningitis.

Classifications:

Exposure: Positive recent contact with suspected or confirmed adult with pulmonary TB, negative PPD, normal physical examination (PE), and normal chest X ray.

Infection: Positive PPD in client with normal PE and normal chest X ray or chest X ray with granuloma or calcifications only.

Disease: Positive PPD, signs and symptoms of disease, and positive chest X ray.

Isolation. Most children who are hospitalized require only standard precautions. Those with positive acid-fast bacillus (AFB) in sputum smears should have airborne precautions until after treatment is effective, sputum shows decreasing organisms, and cough is going away.

Nursing Care. Appropriate testing and interpretation. Isolation if necessary. Administer medication as indicated and educate caregivers of importance of compliance with preventive chemotherapy. Preventive chemotherapy usually with isoniazid (INH) 10 mg/kg/day for 6–9 mo q.d. (max. dose: 300 mg). Those with active disease treated with 6-, 9-, or 12-mo regimens, depending on site of infection, using combination of two, three, or four of the following drugs: INH, rifampin, pyrazinamide, or streptomycin. Partial treatment can lead to drug resistance. All children with active TB should be tested for HIV. Ensure nutritious meals and adequate rest and monitor growth and development.

Complications. Drug resistance; adverse reactions to drug therapy

CONGENITAL CARDIAC DEFECTS AND REPAIRS

Presenting signs and symptoms (depending on defect); degree of the following may vary.

History

Poor feeding, decreased weight gain, tiring with feeding, sweating, frequent respiratory infections, fast or hard breathing, inability to keep up with peers, easily fatigued

Physical Examination

Tachycardia, bradycardia, tachypnea, elevated BP, palpable thrills, decreased pulses, poor perfusion, murmurs; may show symptoms of failure to thrive and lags in development

Work-up

Chest X ray	To determine heart size and location
Electrocardiogram (ECG)	To measure electrical activity of heart
Holter monitor	24-hr monitoring of heart rate (HR) and rhythm
Echocardiogram (ECHO)	Sound waves show images of heart formations
Cardiac catheterization	Catheter is advanced, usually through femoral vessels, to visualize heart structures and blood flow patterns and to measure pressures and oxygen levels

Common Defects and Repairs

Defects Causing Increase in Pulmonary Blood Flow

Atrial Septal Defect (ASD). Opening between atriums. Usually repaired with surgical Dacron patch closure.

Ventricular Septal Defect (VSD). Opening between ventricles. Can be classified as membranous or muscular. Commonly associated with other defects. Small VSDs repaired with pursestring suture, large ones with knitted Dacron patch. Many small VSDs close spontaneously in first year of life.

Endocardial Cushion Defect (Arteriovenous [AV] Canal). Low ASD continuous with high VSD and cleft of mitral and tricuspid valves. Palliative treatment is to do a pulmonary artery (PA) banding. Full repair involves patch closure of septal defects and reconstruction of valve tissue. Some need mitral valve replacements.

Patent Ductus Arteriosus (PDA). Condition in which fetal ductus does not close at birth. Can be treated by surgical ligation, with clip closure, or sometimes occluded during heart catheterization.

Obstructive Defects

Coarctation of Aorta (CoA). Narrowing of aorta at insertion of ductus arteriosus. Surgical repair involves resection with end-to-end anastomosis of aorta or enlargement of constricted section with graft.

Aortic Stenosis (AS). Narrowing or stricture of aortic valve. Can lead to hypertrophy of left ventricle. Treated surgically with aortic valvotomy or valve replacement. Sometimes can dilate narrowed valve with balloon angioplasty in catheterization laboratory (cath. lab.)

Pulmonary Stenosis (PS). Narrowing of entrance to pulmonary artery that can lead to right ventricular hypertrophy. *Pulmonary atresia* is a fused valve that allows no blood flow to lungs and can cause hypoplastic right ventricle. Treated with balloon angioplasty in cath. lab. or transventricular valvotomy (Brock procedure).

Defects Causing Decrease in Pulmonary Blood Flow

Tetralogy of Fallot (TOF). Consists of four major problems: VSD, PS, overriding aorta, and right ventricular hypertrophy. Palliative treatment with Blalock-Taussig (BT) shunt or modified BT shunt to provide pulmonary blood flow from right or left subclavian arteries. Complete repair preferred and involves closure of VSD, resection of stenosis, and pericardial patch.

Tricuspid Atresia. Failure of tricuspid valve to develop. Palliative treatment is placement of pulmonary-to-systemic shunt to increase blood flow to lungs and a second stage of bidirectional Glenn shunt. Repair done with modified Fontan procedure.

Mixed Defects

Transposition of Great Arteries (TGA) or Transposition of Great Vessels (TGV). Pulmonary artery arises from left ventricle and aorta from right, so there is no communication between systemic and pulmonary circulation. Is incompatible with life without associated mixed defects such as PDA, ASD, or VSD. Palliative treatment with prostaglandin to keep PDA open and with balloon atrial septostomy (Rashkind procedure). Surgical repair involves arterial switch within first weeks of life or Senning procedure with intraatrial baffle using atrial septum. Mustard procedure using prosthetic material can be done with older children. Rastelli procedure used when child has TGA, VSD, and severe PS.

Total Anomalous Pulmonary Venous Connection (TAPVC). Pulmonary veins do not join left atrium. Surgical treatment varies with anatomic defect.

Truncus Arteriosus. Pulmonary artery and aorta did not separate and they override both ventricles. Treated with modified Rastelli procedure.

Hypoplastic Left Heart Syndrome (HLHS). Underdevelopment of left side of heart leading to hypoplastic left ventricle and aortic atresia. Surgical treatment with multiple-stage Norwood procedure or heart transplant during newborn period.

Nursing Care

Preoperative

Assess vital signs and exercise tolerance and provide adequate nutrition and rest. May need to increment care to conserve child's energy. Maintain hydration. Assess for signs and symptoms of CHF: tachycardia, diaphoresis, decreased perfusion, cold extremities, mottling, duskiness, tachypnea >60, retractions, cyanosis, orthopnea, cough, wheezing, failure to thrive, hepatomegaly, edema, and/or abnormal weight gain. Assess development. Teach caregivers how to care for child at home or to prepare for surgery if imminent. Provide comfort; administer diuretics and cardiac medications as ordered. Neutral temperature environment conserves energy. If postcatheterization, observe for bleeding and assess circulation of involved extremity.

Postoperative

Assess vital signs. Provide for rest and comfort (administer pain medications as ordered), encourage intake of fluids and progressive ambulation, and give emotional support. Observe for the following complications:

Infection—fever; foul-smelling drainage; increased pain
CHF—signs and symptoms described previously
Cardiac tamponade—Narrowing pulse pressure; tachycardia; dyspnea; cyanosis; apprehension; tripod position
Heart block—usually bradycardia
Post–pericardial syndrome (PPS)—fever; chest pain; irritability

Prepare for discharge by teaching caregiver how to care for child at home and encourage normalcy.

CONJUNCTIVITIS

Brief Description

Inflammation of conjunctiva is termed *conjunctivitis,* also known as *pink eye*. Etiology usually bacterial, viral, allergic, or chemical.

History and Physical Assessment Findings

Examination of external eye reveals diffuse redness of conjunctiva more obvious on palpebral surface. Associated watery or purulent discharge, which usually results in crusting of eyelids, especially on wakening. Child reports minimal pain and normal vision. There is normal papillary and red reflexes.

Nursing Care

Goal is to keep eye(s) clean. Ophthalmic medications need to be administered correctly. Topical antibiotic ointment and/or drops usually prescribed. Accumulated secretions are removed by warm normal saline cleaning. Infection highly contagious via direct contact. (Strict handwashing and keeping child out of school or day care for 24 hr will help minimize transmission.) Systemic antihistamines prescribed for children with allergic conjunctivitis.

Related Nursing Diagnoses

- Infection

CROUP

Brief Description

Croup is a term applied to several viral and bacterial syndromes; however, the most common cause of acute stridor in young children is viral laryngotracheobronchitis (LTB). This upper airway illness results from swelling of structures in the airway and can result in significant airway obstruction. Common pathogens include parainfluenza, RSV, adenovirus, and influenza A. Croup usually occurs in late fall and winter months and incidence peaks at age 6 mo to 3 yr.

History and Physical Assessment Findings

Children with croup have characteristic seal-like, barking cough. Other common symptoms include fever, tachypnea, inspiratory stridor, cough, and hoarseness. Chest X ray may demonstrate steeple sign (i.e., subglottic narrowing). Children with croup may have retractions, mental status changes (especially agitation and restlessness), cyanosis, and low oxygen-saturation levels.

Nursing Care

Imperative to keep child and family calm. This will help facilitate breathing and oxygenation. Humidification and supplemental oxygen (if saturation <92%) therapy common interventions. Corticosteroids (e.g., dexamethasone) may be prescribed to decrease airway edema. Nebulized racemic epinephrine and oral dexamethasone usually prescribed for moderated croup. Children with severe croup usually prescribed nebulized racemic epinephrine and PO/NG prednisolone. Most children with croup managed at home unless respiratory distress severe and warrants frequent monitoring.

Related Nursing Diagnoses

- Ineffective breathing pattern
- Impaired gas exchange
- Fear
- Anxiety
- Deficient knowledge
- Risk for deficient fluid volume

CYSTIC FIBROSIS (CF)

Brief Description

CF is an inherited autosomal-recessive disorder of the exocrine glands, which causes glands to produce highly viscous secretions of mucus. Respiratory, gastrointestinal (GI), musculoskeletal, reproductive, and integumentary systems are altered. Ultimately, all organs with mucous ducts become obstructed and damaged. Is a lack of secretion of enzymes from blocked pancreatic ducts leading to altered digestion of fats and proteins. Lungs become filled with mucus, causing air trapping in small airways and eventually leading to recurrent respiratory infections. Males with CF become sterile because of blockage of vas deferens. Females usually experience infertility resulting from increased mucous secretions in reproductive tract, interfering with sperm mobility.

History and Physical Assessment Findings

History of meconium ileus or other obstructive bowel diseases may be present in infant. Often these are first indications of CF. Fatty stool, termed *steatorrhea*, is a classic sign of CF. Other common signs and symptoms are chronic/productive cough and frequent respiratory infection. Child often has symptoms of failure to thrive despite strong appetite and commonly falls off growth curve. Definitive diagnosis made through skin sweat testing (pilocarpine iontophoresis), presence of aforementioned symptoms, or family history.

Nursing Care

Nursing care centered on the following activities: maintaining respiratory function, managing/preventing infection, ensuring optimum nutrition, preventing GI blockages, and meeting child's and family's psychosocial needs. Nebulized bronchodilators (e.g., albuterol), aerosol dornase alfa, anti-inflammatory agents (e.g., steroids, nonsteroidal anti-inflammatory drugs [NSAIDs]), chest physiotherapy, antibiotics, pancreatic enzyme supplements, multivitamin supplements, and dietary supplements are mainstays of treatment. Because of need for frequent hospitalization, it is important to include caregivers in child's care as much as possible to help maintain child's home routine. Emotional support essential because this disease affects all members of the family and places constraints on daily activities of all involved.

Related Nursing Diagnoses

- Ineffective airway clearance
- Risk for infection
- Imbalanced nutrition: less than body requirements
- Interrupted family processes

DEPRESSION

Brief Description

Children most at risk for depression are those with depressed caregivers, divorced caregivers, hospitalized siblings, attention deficit disorder (ADD)/ADHD, mild mental retardation, low socioeconomic status, and chronic illness. Classic presentation is child who appears sad; however, depression in children may manifest as hyperactivity and aggression.

History and Physical Assessment Findings

Symptoms often include depressed mood, loss of interest, significant weight loss or gain, insomnia or hypersomnia, fatigue, feelings of worthlessness, inappropriate guilt, decreased concentration, and recurrent thoughts of death.

Nursing Care

Seriously depressed children (especially those with suicidal or homicidal ideation) require hospitalization. Outpatient therapy indicated for those with mild to moderate depression. Referral to mental health professional necessary. Psychotherapy and/or pharmacotherapy often indicated.

Related Nursing Diagnoses

- Fatigue
- Risk for disturbed sleep pattern
- Hopelessness
- Social isolation
- Risk for self-directed violence
- Risk for other-directed violence

DERMATITIS

Brief Description

Atopic dermatitis refers to a type of eczema. This skin disorder usually associated with allergy and begins during infancy. Erythema, edema, papules, weeping, scales, and intense pruritus are hallmarks of eczema. *Contact dermatitis* refers to inflammatory skin reaction to chemical substances resulting in hypersensitivity response. Contact dermatitis characterized by acute onset of pruritic papulovesicular lesions localized to site of antigen contact. Common causes include poison ivy/oak/sumac and nickel allergy (from jewelry).

History and Physical Assessment Findings

Atopic dermatitis findings include erythematous papules and vesicles with weeping, oozing, and crusts. Lesions usually found on scalp, forehead, cheeks, forearms, wrists, elbows, and backs of knees. Lesions associated with paroxysmal and intense pruritus. Family history of allergies common (e.g., asthma, hayfever).

Contact dermatitis develops first as early erythema followed by swelling, urticaria, or maculopapular vesicles and scales. Often accompanied by intense pruritus.

Nursing Care

Atopic dermatitis: Goals of management include relieving pruritus, hydrating skin, reducing inflammation, and preventing secondary infection. Cool, wet compresses soothing to skin. Aveeno oatmeal baths useful in relieving pruritus. Antihistamines such as hydroxyzine hydrochloride (Atarax) and diphenhydramine hydrochloride (Benadryl) may also be prescribed. Skin emollients such as Eucerin cream often used to hydrate skin. Families should be instructed to avoid hot baths and scented soaps. Topical steroids such as hydrocortisone ointment, triamcinolone, or fluocinonide (Lidex) may be ordered. Fingernails should be kept short and clean to prevent infection. Lesions should be examined for signs of infection (honey-colored crusting with surrounding erythema) and reported to health care practitioner.

Contact dermatitis: Teach client regarding need to avoid further contact with allergen. Topical steroid preparations usually ordered. Oral antihistamines may be prescribed to alleviate itching. Oral steroids (e.g., prednisone) usually ordered if lesions are on face or genitals, if they are widespread, or if there is generalized edema. Fingernails should be kept short and clean to prevent infection. Lesions should be examined for signs of infection (e.g., increased erythema, linear streaking) and reported to health care practitioner.

Related Nursing Diagnoses

- Impaired skin integrity
- Pain
- Risk for infection
- Risk for disturbed body image
- Deficient knowledge

EATING DISORDERS ANOREXIA NERVOSA

Brief Description

Anorexia nervosa (AN) is characterized by refusal to maintain minimally normal body weight. Is usually significant fear of being overweight. Child experiences hunger but denies it. More prevalent in middle- and upper-class white females. Mean age of onset 13–14 yr. Often described as perfectionists and high achievers. Have disturbed perception of body size even when significantly underweight. Most often, AN presents as lifelong problem.

History and Physical Assessment Findings

Symptoms include weight loss of >15% body weight, amenorrhea, sleep disturbances, denial of illness, arrested pubertal progression, obvious cachexia, hypothermia, bradycardia, hypotension, scalp hair loss, electrolyte imbalances, and ECG abnormalities.

Nursing Care

Outpatient treatment usually recommended for those who have had the disease <4 mo. Family functioning should be intact for those receiving outpatient treatment. Those with severe weight loss, starvation, drug use, abnormal ECG, or severe depression should receive inpatient treatment. Interdisciplinary care with mental health professionals, health care practitioners, social workers, nurses, and nutritionists is necessary. Nutritional therapy, psychotherapy, and/or behavior therapy regimens are used.

Related Nursing Diagnoses

- Ineffective health maintenance
- Imbalanced nutrition: less than body requirements
- Risk for deficient fluid volume
- Hypothermia
- Risk for delayed growth and development
- Disturbed thought processes
- Chronic low self-esteem
- Disturbed body image
- Ineffective individual coping
- Risk for interrupted family processes

EATING DISORDERS
BULIMIA

Brief Description

Bulimia nervosa (BN) is a disorder characterized by binge eating in association with self-induced vomiting, severe food restriction, cathartic or laxative abuse, strenuous exercise, and/or heightened concern with body shape. Binge eaters usually unaware of being hungry before eating but cannot stop once they start. Classified as a type of addiction. Episodes of binging and purging accompanied by depressed mood and awareness of abnormal eating pattern. Those with career aspirations that require low weight (e.g., athletics, modeling) are most at risk.

History and Physical Assessment Findings

History usually reveals that disorder began with only occasional episodes of binging and purging. With progression of disease, frequency of binging and purging and amount of food intake increases; loss of control over behaviors is gradual. Frequency of binging and purging varies from 1x/wk to many times per day. Fluid and electrolyte loss common. May also have diminished reflexes secondary to potassium depletion and cardiac arrhythmias. Laboratory tests often reveal anemia. Erosion of tooth enamel, dental caries, esophagitis, sore throat, and parotitis often findings related to repeated self-induced vomiting and irritation from stomach acid. Backs of hands may be scarred and/or cut from teeth during self-induced vomiting.

Nursing Care

Management of BN involves medical, psychologic, behavioral, and nutritional components. Hospitalization required for those with fluid and electrolyte imbalances and cardiac complications. Outpatient therapy involves nutritional consultation and behavioral therapy. Psychopharmacologic interventions have been effective in reducing urge to binge and vomit. Home environment should be structured so as to reduce potential for binging behavior; includes eliminating binge-type foods (e.g., high-calorie sweets) and restricting eating to one room in the home. Telephone support has been demonstrated to be useful.

Related Nursing Diagnoses

- Ineffective health maintenance
- Imbalanced nutrition: less than body requirements
- Impaired dentition
- Risk for deficient fluid volume
- Chronic low self-esteem
- Disturbed body image
- Risk for self-mutilation
- Interrupted family processes
- Ineffective individual coping

EPIGLOTTITIS

Brief Description

Epiglottitis is an inflammation of the epiglottis and constitutes a pediatric emergency. Edema in this area of the airway can progress rapidly, leading to airway obstruction by occlusion of trachea and epiglottis. Causative organism is often *H. influenzae* type B (Hib). Incidence has decreased since advent of Hib vaccine. Affects children from 6 mo to 10 yr of age (average age is 3 yr old).

History and Physical Assessment Findings

History usually consistent with previously healthy child who *suddenly* becomes ill. Usually report of fever, sore throat, muffled/hoarse voice, and swallowing difficulty. Stridor worsens as larynx swells. Child often observed drooling and assumes tripod (i.e., leaning forward with jaw thrusted forward) posture refusing to lay down. X ray reveals enlarged epiglottis and narrowed airway. Positive blood culture found in most clients with epiglottitis.

Nursing Care

Airway management, medication administration, hydration, and support are vital aspects of care. *Visual inspection of the mouth and throat contraindicated because irritation and hypersensitivity of the airway can lead to laryngospasm.* Emergency equipment for intubation and airway maintenance should be readily available. Child should be kept calm. Children with epiglottitis initially managed in pediatric intensive care unit. IV antibiotics (e.g., cefotaxime, ceftriaxone) given to treat infection, and IV fluids administered to provide hydration.

Related Nursing Diagnoses

- Infection
- Risk for injury
- Impaired gas exchange
- Fear
- Anxiety

GASTROESOPHAGEAL REFLUX (GER)

Brief Description

GER involves the passive return of stomach contents into the esophagus. This results from increased relaxation of the lower esophageal sphincter. Factors that cause this relaxation include gastric distension, coughing, and obstructive lung disease. This disorder results in passive vomiting and may lead to complications such as pneumonia (especially in young infants), apnea (especially in young infants), esophagitis, and midepigastric pain.

History and Physical Assessment Findings

History usually reveals report of passive emesis after feedings. Child may demonstrate poor weight gain (fall off growth curve) in more severe cases. Child may have anemia as result of bleeding from esophageal mucosa. History of multiple respiratory infections should alert you to the possibility of GER. A barium swallow may demonstrate reflux following swallowing. Esophageal pH monitoring positive if pH acidic.

Nursing Care

Small, frequent feedings with thickened formula (rice cereal, 1 tsp/1 oz formula) recommended. Maintenance of prone, elevated position after feeding also recommended. Scientific research regarding effectiveness of these interventions still inconclusive, although this remains the standard in practice.

Pharmacologic agents such as H_2-blockers and prokinetic medications may be prescribed, especially in children with poor weight gain and/or frequent respiratory infection. Surgical treatment reserved for very severe cases.

Related Nursing Diagnoses

- Imbalanced nutrition: less than body requirements
- Risk for injury
- Ineffective health maintenance
- Deficient knowledge

HIRSCHSPRUNG'S DISEASE

Brief Description

Also known as congenital aganglionic megacolon, *Hirschsprung's disease* is a mechanical intestinal obstruction caused by inadequate motility. Ganglionic cells are absent in one or more segments of the colon. Usually involves rectum and large intestine. Lack of enervation causes functional defect, and there is lack of peristalsis, which causes accumulation of bowel contents and distension. Ischemia may occur with resulting enterocolitis, which can lead to death.

History and Physical Assessment Findings

In neonates, history of not passing meconium often found. Neonate may also refuse fluids. Infants generally portray history of failure to thrive, constipation, and abdominal distension. Symptoms during childhood more chronic in nature and include constipation, ribbon-like stools, and visible peristalsis. Medical diagnosis confirmed by X ray, barium enema, and rectal biopsy.

Nursing Care

Medical treatment usually involves surgery to remove aganglionic portion of colon. Temporary colostomy often performed to relieve obstruction. Ostomy usually closed during second surgery when aganglionic portion is removed.

Because enterocolitis is potential complication, vital signs should be monitored frequently to assess for signs of shock. Fluids and electrolytes often replaced. Bowel assessments should be performed to detect symptoms of perforation (e.g., fever, increasing distension, irritablility, vomiting). Abdominal girth measurements often performed to detect progressing distension.

Related Nursing Diagnoses

- Risk for injury
- Imbalanced nutrition: less than body requirements
- Deficient knowledge

IMPETIGO

Brief Description

Impetigo is a highly contagious bacterial infection of the skin. *S. aureus* is most common causative organism. Vesicular-type lesion that spreads peripherally in sharply marginated irregular outlines. Tends to heal without scarring unless secondary infections occur. Easily spread by self-inoculation, and therefore children should be advised to avoid touching involved area. Most common in infants and young children.

History and Physical Assessment Findings

Be alert to history of lesions that begin as red macules and then become vesicular. Lesions are moist vesicles that rupture to form thick, honey-colored crusting. Most commonly located around mouth and nose. Pruritus is common. Child usually asymptomatic; systemic effects are minimal.

Nursing Care

Topical antibiotic cream (e.g., mupirocin [Bactroban]) may be prescribed. Topical treatment usually prescribed for 1 wk to 10 days. Children who have widespread lesions and are systemically ill may be prescribed oral antibiotics (e.g., cephalexin or cloxacillin). Area should be gently cleansed with warm water. Caregivers should be taught about highly contagious nature of this infection. Other family members should be assessed.

Related Nursing Diagnoses

- Impaired skin integrity
- Pain
- Risk for infection
- Deficient knowledge

INSULIN-DEPENDENT DIABETES MELLITUS (IDDM)

Brief Description

IDDM is the most common chronic metabolic disorder in children. IDDM (also called *type I diabetes*) results in hyperglycemia usually secondary to insulin deficiency. Is loss of pancreas β-cell functioning and insulin production. Result is chronic high blood sugar and other problems with carbohydrate and fat metabolism. Mode of inheritance still not well described. Some evidence suggests that genetic predisposition is important factor. Viral infection thought to be significant antecedent. This type of antecedent thought to initiate autoimmune process that gradually destroys β-cells.

Diabetic ketoacidosis (DKA) is a metabolic state characterized by acidosis, elevated serum glucose, and serum ketones. DKA may be precipitated by physical or emotional stress, infection, and noncompliance with insulin therapy. Often, first presentation of IDDM in children is DKA.

History and Physical Assessment Findings

History generally reveals weight loss, polydipsia, polyphagia, and polyuria. Other physical examination findings usually within normal limits unless child is in DKA. Children in DKA appear weak and lethargic, progressing to comatose. Signs and symptoms of severe dehydration often present. Breath may have fruity odor and Kussmaul's respirations may be present. Laboratory tests demonstrate elevated fasting blood sugar and postprandial glucose levels. Oral glucose tolerance test (OGTT) may be ordered to confirm diagnosis.

Nursing Care

Multidisciplinary focus of care necessary (i.e., involving endocrinologist, diabetes nurse educator, nutritionist, social worker, school nurse). Insulin therapy is hallmark of treatment. Children generally prescribed two daily doses of SC insulin (regular and intermediate or long-acting types). More intensive insulin dosages (>2 injections of continuous SC infusion via insulin pump) may be prescribed. Child and caregivers are taught about insulin administration (e.g., mixing insulins, injection sites). Urine ketones monitored if glucose levels are >250 mg/dL or if child is sick.

Children and families also taught how to perform self blood glucose monitoring. Diet counseling required; consistency of meal times is paramount concern. Exercise is promoted. Signs, symptoms, and treatment of hypoglycemia taught to caregivers and children. Psychologic support to assist in coping with this lifelong chronic illness necessary.

Treating children with DKA considered medical emergency. Fluids replaced IV. Important not to administer fluids too quickly to minimize risk of cerebral edema. IV regular insulin administered at rate of 0.1 U/kg/hr. Glucose levels monitored frequently. Bicarbonate may be prescribed in children who are acidotic. Frequent monitoring of vital signs and intake and output required. ECG monitoring used to detect arrhythmias related to potassium imbalance.

Related Nursing Diagnoses

- Risk for injury
- Deficient knowledge
- Deficient fluid volume
- Interrupted family processes
- Ineffective health maintenance
- Risk for noncompliance

IRON DEFICIENCY ANEMIA

Brief Description

Inadequate supply of dietary iron is the most common cause of *iron deficiency anemia.* Is most prevalent nutritional disorder in the United States. Both young children and adolescents are at risk. Major decrease in incidence has been linked to programs such as Women, Infants, and Children (WIC), although is still a major health problem in children, especially those from low-income families. Other causes of iron deficiency anemia include impaired absorption of iron, blood loss, excessive demands for iron, and inability to form hemoglobin.

History and Physical Assessment Findings

Signs and symptoms of iron deficiency anemia most often not obvious. Some common signs are low weight, paleness, tachycardia, positive guaiac test, poor muscle development, and "spoon" nail. History often reveals increased ingestion of milk. Blood analyses reveal hypochromic, microcytic red blood cells (RBCs); low mean corpuscular volume (MCV) and mean corpuscular hemoglobin concentration (MCHC); low reticulocyte count; and low serum ferritin.

Nursing Care

Aim of treatment is to correct cause of anemia. Most often involves dietary counseling. Oral iron supplements usually prescribed. Important to assess compliance with medication administration. Caregivers should be taught proper administration techniques, which include avoiding administration with milk or other products high in phosphorus.

Related Nursing Diagnoses

- Imbalanced nutrition: less than body requirements
- Ineffective health maintenance
- Deficient knowledge

LEAD POISONING

Brief Description

Lead in paint is the most common source of lead poisoning in young children. Ingestion of contaminated food, water, and soil can also lead to lead exposure. African-American children living in inner cities represent largest number of children with lead poisoning. Children absorb and retain more lead proportionately to their weight than adults, putting them at greater risk of poisoning.

History and Physical Assessment Findings

History usually reveals environmental exposure to lead. Clinical manifestations will vary depending on lead level. Children with lead poisoning may be asymptomatic. However, those with moderate to high lead levels may demonstrate learning or behavior problems, irritability, anorexia, malaise, headache, abdominal pain, and vomiting. Those with severe lead poisoning may experience clumsiness, encephalopathy, coma, convulsions, and signs of increased IP.

Nursing Care

Interventions aimed at removing sources of lead in child's environment necessary. Treatment consists of chelation therapy as agents bind with lead leading to increased excretion. Agents such as calcium disodium ethylenediaminetetraacetic acid ($CaNa_2$ EDTA), dimercaprol (BAL), and D-penicillamine or dimercaptosuccinic acid (DMSA) often used. Nursing care should also be aimed at screening, prevention, and education. Caregivers need to understand importance of follow-up testing. Home health care referrals and/or social work referral may be appropriate.

Related Nursing Diagnoses

- Risk for injury
- Imbalanced nutrition: less than body requirements
- Ineffective health maintenance
- Risk for constipation
- Disturbed sensory perception
- Risk for impaired parenting

OBSESSIVE-COMPULSIVE DISORDER (OCD)

Brief Description

OCD is characterized by repetitive actions that the child knows are abnormal. Often, repetitive handwashing or certain words said before performing a task are symptoms exhibited by the child. Children with OCD may have obsessive thoughts about fear of harm, illness, death, and wrongdoing.

History and Physical Assessment Findings

Classic sign of OCD is child's understanding that the repetitive actions are abnormal and thoughts irrational.

Nursing Care

Management of child with OCD involves behavior modification, psychopharmacologic intervention, and psychotherapy.

Related Nursing Diagnoses

- Fatigue
- Disturbed thought processes
- Ineffective individual coping

ORBITAL CELLULITIS

Brief Description

Orbital cellulitis is the infection of orbital contents posterior to orbital septum. Usually spreads from adjacent infection of sinus. Common organisms are *S. aureus*, group A streptococci, *S. pneumoniae*, and *H. influenzae* type B.

History and Physical Assessment Findings

Symptoms often include obvious lid edema, pain on eye movement, decreased ocular mobility, and decreased visual acuity. History often reveals sinus congestion/infection.

Nursing Care

Patient hospitalized for IV antibiotics. Ophthalmology referral should be made. Cultures should be obtained. Child needs to be prepared for computed tomography (CT) scan of orbit and sinus. Surgical intervention may be necessary. Need to assess for signs and symptoms of meningeal irritation because risk of bacterial meningitis is increased in those with orbital cellulitis.

Related Nursing Diagnoses

- Infection
- Pain
- Disturbed sensory perception

OSTEOMYELITIS

Brief Description

Osteomyelitis represents an infection of the bone. Any bone can be affected but femoral and tibial metaphyses most commonly involved. Results from either hematogenous spread (preexisting infection elsewhere) or exogenous (invasion of bone from outside body). Common pathogens are *S. aureus*, group A streptococci, *H. influenzae, Pseudomonas* organisms, and *Salmonella* organisms.

History and Physical Assessment Findings

Child may have history of trauma or fever. Often report limp or inability to bear weight. Affected limb looks swollen, bruised, red, hot, and tender. Child often febrile and irritable and appears systemically ill. Laboratory tests reveal elevated WBCs and erythrocyte sedimentation rate (ESR). Positive blood culture and positive culture of aspirate from involved bone.

Nursing Care

One of the first priorities of care is prompt administration of IV antibiotics. Antibiotic therapy usually indicated for several weeks. Caregivers may be taught home administration using a central venous catheter. Child maintained on bed rest with affected extremity immobilized (may need splint or cast). Bed rest and immobilization help prevent spread of infection. Surgical interventions may be required in certain cases. Positioning and comfort measures necessary. Physical therapy consult often initiated as child begins to increase mobility.

Related Nursing Diagnoses

- Pain
- Infection
- Hyperthermia
- Ineffective tissue perfusion: bone
- Impaired mobility
- Interrupted family processes

OTITIS MEDIA

Brief Description

OM is an inflammation of the middle ear. Represents one of the most prevalent diseases in young children. Results from dysfunctioning eustachian tube and often is first childhood illness confronted by caregivers.

Incidence greatest in children age 6 mo to 2 yr and is higher in winter months. Children exposed to ETS also have higher incidence. *S. pneumoniae* and *H. influenzae* are most common pathogens. Viral agents identified in approximately 40% of cases.

History and Physical Assessment Findings

Otoscopic examination reveals red tympanic membrane (often bulging) with no visible landmarks. History reveals ear pain as evidenced by pulling on ear, fever, irritability, poor PO intake, and/or associated upper respiratory infection.

Nursing Care

A variety of antibiotics are used to treat OM. Amoxicillin remains first-line drug. Compliance by caregiver and child with antibiotic administration should be assessed. Other commonly prescribed antibiotics are amoxicillin/clavulanate (Augmentin), cefixime (Suprax), erythromycin (Pediazole), cefuroxime (Ceftin), and cotrimoxazole (Bactrim). Analgesics/antipyretics such as Tylenol and Motrin are also used to treat fever and/or discomfort. Decongestants and antihistamines have not proven effective.

Related Nursing Diagnoses

- Pain
- Infection
- Disturbed sensory perception

PEDICULOSIS CAPITIS (HEAD LICE)

Brief Description

Pediculosis capitis is a parasitic infection of the scalp by the louse. Lice infestations are highly communicable. Eggs or nits are at junction of hair shaft close to skin. Head lice are spread by hair-to-hair contact, clothing, and brushes. Louse cannot fly and is transmitted from person to person via personal items. Child may have psychologic effects because infection can be highly stressful to child and family.

History and Physical Assessment Findings

Scalp pruritus with erythema and excoriations common. Live lice and nits may be seen on hair shaft. Lice are visible to the naked eye as small, grayish dots. Nits appear as whitish specks visible approximately 1/4 inch from scalp and may look like dandruff.

Nursing Care

Pediculicides such as Kwell shampoo often prescribed. Nix cream rinse may be purchased over the counter and has shown to be more effective and safer than Kwell in children. Manual removal of nits with fine-tooth comb also necessary. Care of environment necessary (e.g., washing clothing and bed linens in hot water, vacuuming carpets, boiling hair-care items for 10 min). Children should be taught not to share hair-care items such as combs and barrettes nor caps and other items worn near hair.

Related Nursing Diagnoses

- Infection
- Deficient knowledge
- Interrupted family processes
- Situational low self-esteem

PNEUMONIA

Brief Description

Pneumonia is an infection and inflammation of the lower respiratory tract, specifically of the bronchioles and alveolar spaces of the lungs. Etiology may be viral, bacterial, or mycoplasmal. End-result of pathogen invasion results in accumulation of exudates, which fill alveolar spaces, and consolidation of lung areas.

History and Physical Assessment Findings

History may include acute or subacute onset of symptoms. Symptoms of fever (with chills), cough, dyspnea, tachypnea, shallow breathing, and rales common. X-ray findings of consolidation confirm diagnosis, although most children diagnosed by clinical symptoms. CBC results reveal elevated WBCs.

Nursing Care

Most children managed at home but inpatient therapy required for those with significant infection and respiratory distress. Ongoing respiratory assessments indicated. Prescription of anti-infectives depends on type of pneumonia. Pain management may be necessary, especially during coughing and deep breathing. Antipyretics may be necessary to control fever. Providing adequate hydration also priority of care.

Related Nursing Diagnoses

- Infection
- Impaired gas exchange

- Ineffective airway clearance
- Ineffective health maintenance

POST-TRAUMATIC STRESS DISORDER (PTSD)

Brief Description

Children with PTSD have a history of exposure to an adverse event thought to be distressing to nearly everyone. Trauma may be persistently reexperienced. Often, these types of events include life-threatening events to self or significant others; death of a loved one; serious injury; physical coercion; an accident; assault; disasters (e.g., flood, plane crash, hurricane); sexual abuse; and/or witnessing homicide, suicide, or shooting. Risk for PTSD higher in children who experience more than one of these events.

History and Physical Assessment Findings

Children with PTSD often report difficulty with sleeping, nightmares, anxiety, difficulty with interpersonal relationships, phobias, and agitation.

Nursing Care

Children who experience any traumatic event need to learn how to deal with their emotions. Type of management depends on intensity of event and individual reactions to it. Often, psychologic intervention by mental health professional is necessary.

Related Nursing Diagnoses

- Hopelessness
- Ineffective individual coping
- Posttrauma syndrome
- Interrupted family processes
- Risk for other-directed violence
- Dysfunctional grieving

SCOLIOSIS

Brief Description

Scoliosis is a lateral curvature of the spine. Most cases idiopathic in nature because there is no apparent cause, but there are also congenital and neuromuscular causes. Most common spinal deformity. Girls more commonly affected. Usual age of onset is 10–11 yr.

History and Physical Assessment Findings

Child may complain of clothes not fitting well (e.g., uneven pant length). Otherwise, few obvious signs present at time of diagnosis. Child may exhibit asymmetry of shoulder height, scapula, or hip height. X-ray studies and magnetic resonance imaging (MRI) are primary diagnostic tests used.

Nursing Care

Although controversial, screening programs used with adolescents (by school nurses and at well-child visits). Early management consists of bracing (Boston brace, Milwaukee brace) and supplemental exercises. Noncompliance and body image disturbances common with children who wear braces. Surgical correction (e.g., spinal fusion with Harrington rods, Luque instrumentation, or Cotrel-Dubousset procedure) required for severe curvatures.

Related Nursing Diagnoses

- Risk for injury
- Risk for impaired skin integrity
- Disturbed body image
- Pain
- Impaired physical mobility
- Risk for interrupted family processes

SEIZURES

Brief Description

Seizures represent brief malfunctioning within the brain's electrical system. Abnormal electrical discharges from the brain cause paroxysmal, uncontrolled episodes of behavior. Common causes include CNS bleeding, CNS infection, metabolic abnormalities, head trauma, tumor, toxin ingestion, and fever. Seizures usually idiopathic in nature.

Consequences of seizure activity can include alterations in responsiveness, in sensation and perception, and in movement and muscle tone. Seizures classified as partial (i.e., limited to particular area of brain), generalized (i.e., involve both hemispheres of brain), or unclassified.

History and Physical Assessment Findings

Child and family should be asked to specifically describe seizure. Need to distinguish seizures from breath-holding spells. Careful seizure observation and documentation necessary. Describe beginning of episode including any precipitating factors, including an aura. Also describe child's response to self and others. Clear description of movements, mobility, and tone necessary. Include observation of exact location, indicating whether one or both sides of body are affected. Assessment made for any postictal responses. Note how long it takes for child to resume previous activities. Results of CT scan, MRI, EEG, skull radiography, electromyogram (EMG), brain scan, lumbar puncture, and antiepileptic drug–blood levels should be noted.

Nursing Care

Prompt recognition of seizure activity necessary to ensure safety. Stay with child during seizure. Protect child from potential injury (e.g., falls, aspiration pneumonia, hyperthermia). Be sure not to restrain child's movements. Reorient child after episode while providing reassurance and psychologic support for child and family. Emergency assistance should be sought if there is respiratory arrest or if seizure activity lasts for >5 min (status epilepticus), multiple seizure episodes occur without return of consciousness in between (status epilepticus), or child has sustained injury.

IV or PR administration of antiepileptic drugs such as diazepam, phenytoin, or phenobarbital indicated during episodes of status epilepticus. Children usually are maintained on daily PO dosages of antiepileptic drugs. Client teaching regarding seizures, antiepileptic drugs, diagnostic testing, seizure recognition, and first aid necessary.

Related Nursing Diagnoses

- Risk for injury
- Disturbed sensory perception
- Ineffective health maintenance

SEXUALLY TRANSMITTED DISEASES (STDs)

Chlamydial Infections

Infective Organism. Bacterium *Chlamydia trachomatis*

Sources. Humans

Transmission. Sexual

Incubation Period. 8–21 days

Signs and Symptoms. Urethritis, cervicitis, salpingitis, inguinal lymphadenopathy, vaginal discharge, dysuria, epididymitis, proctitis, lower abdominal pain, and menstrual irregularities. May be totally asymptomatic.

Diagnosis. Cell culture

Nursing Care. PO antibiotics (e.g., doxycycline, azithromycin). Single-dose therapy preferred if possible. All sexual contacts should be treated. Follow-up therapy should be stressed. Reportable in most states.

Complications. Chronic conjunctivitis

Gonorrhea

Infective Organism. *Neisseria gonorrhoeae*, gram-negative diplococcus

Sources. Humans

Transmission. Almost always sexually transmitted except in cases of vertical transmission from maternal cervix to conjunctiva of newborn.

Incubation Period. 2–6 days; in rare cases, 10–16 days

Signs and Symptoms. Large percentage of clients asymptomatic. Clinical signs may include urethritis (males); cervicitis (females); pelvic inflammatory disease (PID); pharyngitis; and systemic complications of arthritis, dermatitis, meningitis, and endocarditis.

Diagnosis. Culture and Gram's stain. Patients with gonorrhea should be screened for other STDs.

Nursing care. Single injection or oral dose of antibiotics (e.g., ceftriaxone or cefixime). All sexual contacts should be treated. Important to stress treatment to prevent longterm complications. Prevention strategies encouraged (e.g., case finding, public health education, use of condoms and spermacide). Mandatory reporting required.

Complications. Genitourinary problems in males, occlusion of fallopian tubes in females, sterility.

Herpes Simplex Virus Type 2 (HSV-2)

Infective Organism. Herpes simplex virus type 2 (HSV-2)

Sources. Humans

Transmission. Through contact with lesions

Incubation Period. 2–12 days

Signs and Symptoms. Presentation ranges from asymptomatic to systemic illness. Single lesion or cluster of papules can appear on genitalia, thighs, and/or buttocks. Papules develop into vesicles and pustules and eventually become ulcerations. Intense pain and itching occur when ulcers break. Area lymph nodes enlarge frequently.

Diagnosis. Viral culture

Nursing care. Acyclovir (PO) is drug of choice. Oral sex should be discouraged if lesions are in mouth or on, lips, vagina, or penis. Anal intercourse should be discouraged when lesions are active. Lesions should be washed with soap and water to prevent secondary infection. Condom use recommended. Immunocompromised clients at risk for systemic infection.

Sexual partners with lesions should be treated. Increased risk for HIV in those with open lesions.

Complications. Encephalitis, herpes simplex keratitis, gingivostomatitis.

Human Papilloma Virus (HPV)

Infective Organism. Human papilloma virus (HPV)

Sources. Humans

Transmission. Sexual contact; precursor to cancer of cervix. Perinatal transmission to infants.

Incubation Period. 1–6 mo

Signs and Symptoms. Condyloma acuminatum (wart with cauliflower-like appearance) located on genitalia, around anus, or in mouth. Size varies from several millimeters to several centimeters.

Diagnosis. Physical examination and viral cultures

Nursing Care. No cure exists. Virus controlled by podofilox or interferon. Warts can be removed by cryotherapy or laser surgery.

Syphilis

Infective Organism. *Spirochaeta pallida/Treponema pallidum*

Sources. Humans

Transmission. Congenital transmission to fetus; otherwise, transmitted sexually

Incubation Period. 10–90 days; most infectious during first year of disease

Signs and Symptoms. Chancre in anogenital region, rash, general malaise, condyloma latum papules on moist areas of skin. Congenital—mucocutaneous lesions, snuffles, hepatosplenomegaly, lymphadenopathy, and failure to thrive. Infant also may be asymptomatic.

Diagnosis. Serologic tests for Venereal Disease Research Laboratory (VDRL) and rapid plasma reagent (RPR)

Nursing Care. Congenital syphilis—penicillin G for 10–14 days. Acquired syphilis—penicillin G IM, doxycycline PO, or tetracycline PO depending on age of child and duration of disease. All sexual partners should be contacted, evaluated, and treated. Clients should have repeat VDRL 3, 6, and 12 mo after therapy. Mandatory reporting required.

SICKLE CELL ANEMIA

Brief Description

Sickle cell anemia is a hereditary hemoglobinopathy in which there is partial or complete replacement of normal hemoglobin with abnormal hemoglobin S. Is an autosomal-recessive disorder. Therefore, if both parents have sickle cell trait, there is 25% chance that offspring will have disease.

Occurs most in those of African descent and occasionally affects people of Mediterranean descent.

Hemoglobin in RBCs acquires an elongated crescent or sickle shape. These cells are more rigid and obstruct capillary blood flow, leading to tissue ischemia. Organs become scarred from damaged tissue. Sickling triggered by events such as fever, stress, dehydration, and hypoxia. Sickled cells resume more normal shape with hydration and oxygenation; however, cell membrane is more fragile and cell life is only 10–20 days versus normal 120 days.

History and Physical Assessment Findings

Symptoms generally do not appear until 4–6 mo of age because of presence of fetal hemoglobin. Diagnosis made by hemoglobin electrophoresis through newborn screening. Results in shortened life span of blood vessels. Also tissue destruction, which results from vaso-occlusion.

Changes occur in most body systems, although most common signs and symptoms include the following:

- Brain—headache; convulsion; visual problems (indicative of cerebrovascular accident)
- Eyes—diminished vision as result of retinopathy; retinal detachment
- Skin—decreased peripheral circulation leading to leg ulcers
- Extremities—peripheral neuropathy; weakness; arthralgia
- Bones—susceptibility to infection as result of chronic ischemia
- Liver—engorgement and scarring
- Spleen—fibrosis of spleen leading to increased number of infections

There are three types of sickle cell crisis:

1. Vaso-occlusive—most common type; painful; caused by stasis of blood with cell clumping in microcirculation, ischemia, infarction; fever, pain, and tissue engorgement are common signs
2. Splenic sequestration—life-threatening crisis; caused by pooling of blood within spleen; anemia, hypovolemia, and shock are common signs
3. Aplastic crisis—reduced production and increased destruction of RBCs; crisis usually triggered by viral infection; anemia and pallor are common signs

Nursing Care

No cure for sickle cell anemia. Nursing care should aim at prevention and treatment of sickling episodes. Prevention strategies include avoiding exposure to infections, maintaining adequate hydration, promptly treating infections, and maintaining routine health visits. For children experiencing sickle cell crises, treatment includes hydration restoration, supplemental oxygenation, pain management, treatment and/or prevention of infection, and bed rest. Children may require blood transfusions to treat anemia.

Related Nursing Diagnoses

- Ineffective tissue perfusion
- Deficient fluid volume
- Pain
- Impaired physical mobility
- Risk for infection
- Risk for injury
- Deficient knowledge
- Interrupted family processes
- Risk for impaired parenting

SLIPPED CAPITAL FEMORAL EPIPHYSIS (SCFE)

Brief Description

SCFE is a displacement (abrupt or gradual) of the proximal femoral epiphysis. Usually develops during accelerated periods of growth (preadolescent and adolescent) and is more common in obese children. Although cause is unknown, SCFE is thought to be influenced by hormonal factors (growth hormone, sex hormones). Also associated with endocrine disorders such as hypothyroidism and growth hormone deficiency.

History and Physical Assessment Findings

Child usually reports limp and acute pain in groin, thigh, or knee. Hip range of motion (ROM) painful and limited. X-ray studies demonstrate altered position of femoral head.

Nursing Care

Assessment of child's ROM, pain, and limp necessary. Before treatment, it is essential that child keep weight off affected joint. Children with SCFE require surgical intervention (fixation with screws or pins). Nursing management requires caring for child in traction, administering analgesics and other pain-reduction interventions, educating child and family about disorder, and promoting compliance with medical regimen.

Related Nursing Diagnoses

- Impaired physical mobility
- Pain

- Risk for disturbed body image
- Risk for imbalanced nutrition: more than body requirements
- Risk for infection
- Ineffective tissue perfusion
- Deficient knowledge

SUBSTANCE ABUSE

Brief Description

Most adolescents have some experience with an illicit drug by the time they are high school seniors. Some of these adolescents progress to dependence. Risk factors include any of the following factors: family history of alcoholism or use of other drugs, history of family conflict, history of physical and/or sexual abuse, antisocial behavior, academic underachievement, low self-esteem, peers who use drugs, and early first use of illicit drugs. Often, substance abuse progresses from use of beer, wine, and tobacco to liquor to marijuana to cocaine or heroin. Many adolescents use multiple drugs simultaneously. Some commonly abused substances include alcohol, marijuana and other cannabis substances, CNS depressants such as barbiturates, CNS stimulants such as amphetamines, cocaine, hallucinogens such as lysergic acid diethylamide (LSD), opioids such as morphine and heroin, and volatile substances such as hydrocarbons and nitrous oxide.

History and Physical Assessment Findings

Be alert to history findings consistent with personality changes, unexplained behavior or behavior out of the ordinary, poor family interaction, deteriorating school performance, and withdrawal from regular activities (e.g., sports, extracurricular activities, church). Injuries related to falls, fights, and motor vehicle accidents also should alert you to the possibility of substance abuse. Majority of youth who attempt suicide have history of many years of substance abuse.

Nursing Care

Treatment of drug toxicity or withdrawal depends on actual drug used. Long-term rehabilitation often requires adolescent to be withdrawn from both the environment and the actual chemical. May involve treatment programs such as Alcoholics Anonymous, Narcotics Anonymous, and other similar 12-step programs. Nurses must also play major role in prevention programs.

Related Nursing Diagnoses

- Ineffective denial
- Ineffective coping

- Powerlessness
- Imbalanced nutrition: less than body requirements
- Sexual dysfunction
- Interrupted family processes
- Risk for self-directed violence
- Risk for other-directed violence
- Chronic low self-esteem

ULCERATIVE COLITIS (UC)

Brief Description

UC is considered a chronic inflammatory bowel disease characterized by exacerbations and remissions. Etiology multifactorial in nature and thought to involve infectious organisms, dietary habits, genetic susceptibility, and environmental toxins. Most severly affected sites are the colon and rectum. Areas become ulcerated and edematous. Continous segments of bowel affected at both mucosa and submucosa layers.

History and Physical Assessment Findings

Symptoms often include bloody diarrhea, intense abdominal pain, and weight loss. Diarrhea often severe. Medical diagnosis based on history, physical findings, laboratory tests (e.g., CBC, sedimentation rate, total protein, albumin), and other diagnostic tests (e.g., upper GI, barium enema, endoscopy).

Nursing Care

Pharmacologic treatment for UC involves drugs that control inflammation. Corticosteroids are most effective medication. Nutritional support paramount concern in children with UC because of growth retardation. Both enteral and parenteral nutritional support may be necessary. Children with UC need well-balanced, high-protein and high-calorie diet. Frequently a need for supplemental multivitamins, iron, and folic acid. Surgery may be indicated in clients who do not respond well to medical and nutritional approaches.

Related Nursing Diagnoses

- Imbalanced nutrition: less than body requirements
- Pain
- Disturbed body image
- Risk for deficient fluid volume
- Risk for infection
- Interrupted family processes

URINARY TRACT INFECTION (UTI)

Brief Description

Urinary tract infection is primarily caused by *Escherichia coli* and other gram-negative enteric pathogens. Other causative pathogens include *Proteus* species, enterococci, *Klebsiella* species, *S. aureus*, and *Pseudomonas* species. Anatomic, physical, and chemical conditions and urinary tract properties are factors that contribute to development of UTI. Urinary stasis is most common host factor. UTIs more commonly seen in females because of short urethra and its proximity to anus.

History and Physical Assessment Findings

Common assessment findings include dysuria, frequency, urgency, costovertebral angle tenderness, and enuresis. Nonspecific findings such as vomiting, diarrhea, fever, and lethargy also may be present. Should be noted that some UTIs are asymptomatic. Positive urine culture confirms diagnosis. Diagnostic tests such as voiding cystourethrogram (VCUG) may be necessary to detect anatomic defects.

Nursing Care

Depending on culture and sensitivity results, specific antibiotics are administered. Penicillins, sulfonamides, cephalosporins, and tetracyclines are most commonly prescribed antibiotics for UTIs. Route of administration usually is PO unless child has pyelonephritis, in which case IV route is used. Antipyretics used to decrease fever. Renal ultrasound and VCUG may be ordered to rule out any anatomic problems after infection is cleared. Child and family may need education regarding prevention (e.g., practicing proper hygiene, avoiding bubble baths, wearing cotton underwear) and treatment of infection.

Related Nursing Diagnoses

- Infection
- Risk for injury
- Pain
- Deficient knowledge

URTICARIA

Brief Description

Urticaria generally represents an allergic response to drugs or infection. May be accompanied by general malaise, fever, and lymphadenopathy.

Severe reactions may involve internal organs and joints. Obstruction of airway constitutes medical emergency. Multiple etiologies, but often cause is not identified. Some common causes are drugs (e.g., penicillin, acetylsalicylic acid), food (e.g., peanuts, milk, shellfish, food additives), insect bites, infection, heat, and animal dander. Urticaria may occur as acute, chronic, or recurrent attack.

History and Physical Assessment Findings

Cause for urticaria often unknown. Family members and child should be questioned regarding exposure to any of previously noted common causes. Lesions usually are circular wheals with well-circumscribed borders, but can be of variable size and shape. Tend to appear quickly. Lesions may be localized or generalized and may include swelling of tongue.

Nursing Care

Antihistamines (e.g., hydroxyzine hydrochloride [Atarax], diphenhydramine hydrochloride [Benadryl]) prescribed for urticaria. If severe, oral prednisone may be prescribed. If clients experience recurrent acute episodes, EpiPen kit (for auto-injection of epinephrine) should be carried. If possible, families should try to identify and avoid allergens.

Related Nursing Diagnoses

- Pain
- Risk for injury
- Deficient knowledge

CHAPTER 7

CLINICAL REFERENCES

PEDIATRIC NURSING JOURNALS

Journal of Pediatric Health Care

National Association of Pediatric Nurse Associates and Practitioners
Mosby
11830 Westline Industrial Drive
St. Louis, MO 63146-3318
1-800-325-4177, ext. 4350

Journal of Pediatric Nursing

Nursing Care of Children and Families
W.B. Saunders Company
6277 Sea Harbor Drive
Orlando, FL 32887-4800
1-407-345-4000

Journal of Pediatric Oncology Nursing

W.B. Saunders Company
6277 Sea Harbor Drive
Orlando, FL 32887-4800
1-407-345-4000

Journal of the Society of Pediatric Nurses

Nursecom
1211 Locust Street
Philadelphia, PA 19107
1-800-242-6757

MCN, The American Journal of Maternal/Child Nursing

Lippincott Williams & Wilkins
16522 Hunters Green Parkway
Hagerstown, MD 21704
1-800-638-3030

Pediatric Nursing

Jannetti Publications, Inc.
East Holly Avenue
Box 56
Pitman, NJ 08071-0056
1-856-256-2300

RESOURCES FOR CHILD-HEALTH NURSING AND TOLL-FREE PHONE NUMBERS

General Child Health Resources

American Academy of Pediatrics
141 Northwest Point Boulevard
Elk Grove Village, IL 60007-1098
1-847-434-4000
http://www.aap.org

Centers for Disease Control and Prevention (CDC)
1600 Clifton Road
Atlanta, GA 30333
1-404-639-3311
http://www.cdc.gov

Information for children and families
http://www.kidshealth.org

National Immunization Hotline (at the CDC)
English 1-800-232-2522
Spanish 1-800-232-0233
http://www.cdc.gov/nip

National Parent to Parent Support and Information System, Inc (NPPSIS)
P.O. Box 907
Blue Ridge, GA 30513
1-800-651-1151

National Safe Kids
http://www.safekids.org

AIDS/HIV Resources

AIDS Information Hotline
English 1-800-342-2437
Spanish 1-800-344-7432
http://www.cdc.gov/hiv/hivinfo/nah.htm

National Pediatric and Family HIV Resource Center
1-800-362-0071
http://www.pedhivaids.org

Asthma Resources

American Academy of Allergy, Asthma, and Immunology
1-800-822-2762
http://www.aaaai.org

Asthma and Allergy Foundation of America
1233 20th Street, NW, Suite 402
Washington, D.C. 20036
1-202-466-7643
http://www.aafa.org

American Lung Association
1-800-586-4872
http://www.lungusa.org

National Heart, Lung, and Blood Institute
National Asthma Education Program
NIH Building 31, Room 4A21
9000 Rockville Pike
Bethesda, MD 20892
1-301-251-1222
http://www.nhlbi.nih.gov/health/public/lung/index.htm#asthma

Birth Defects/Disabled Children Resources

Association of Birth Defects in Children
930 Woodcock Road, Suite 225
Orlando, FL 32803
1-407-245-7035
http://www.birthdefects.org

Blind Children's Center
4120 Marathon Street
Los Angeles, CA 90029-3584
1-800-222-3566
http://www.blindcntr.org/bcc

Deafness Research Foundation
1050 17th Street, NW, Suite 701
Washington, DC 20036
1-202-289-5850
http://drf.org

National Clearing House for Infants with Disabilities and Life-Threatening Conditions
1-800-922-9234 ext. 201
http://www.healthy.net/pan/cso/cioi/nicidltc.htm

March of Dimes Birth Defects Foundation
1275 Mamaroneck Avenue
White Plains, NY 10605
1-888-663-4637
http://www.modimes.org

National Down Syndrome Society
666 Broadway
New York, NY 10012
1-212-460-9330
http://www.ndss.org

National Easter Seals Society for Crippled Children
230 West Monroe Street, Suite 1800
Chicago, IL 60606
1-312-726-6200
http://www.easter-seals.org

United Cerebral Palsy Association
UCP National
1660 L Street NW, Suite 700
Washington, DC 20036-5602
1-800-USA-5UCP
http://www.ucpa.org

Cancer Resources

American Cancer Society
1-800-ACS-2345
http://www.cancer.org

The Leukemia & Lymphoma Society
600 Third Avenue
New York, NY 10016
1-800-955-4572
http://www.leukemia.org

National Cancer Institute
NIH Building 31, Room 10A03
31 Center Drive MSC 2580
Bethesda, MD 20892-2580
1-800-4-CANCER
http://www.nci.nih.gov

Diabetes/Renal Resources

Juvenile Diabetes Foundation International
432 Park Avenue South
New York, NY 10016
1-800-223-1138

National Kidney Foundation
30 East 33rd Street, Suite 1100
New York, NY 10016
1-800-622-9010
http://www.kidney.org

Drug Abuse Resources

National Cocaine Hotline
1-800-COCAINE or 1-800-662-HELP

National Clearing House for Alcohol and Drug Information
1-800-729-6686
http://www.health.org

National Council on Alcoholism and Drug Dependence
12 W. 21st Street
New York, NY 10010
1-800-622-2255

National Institute of Drug Abuse
6001 Executive Boulevard
Bethesda, MD 20892-9561
1-301-443-1124

Heart Disease Resources

American Heart Association
National Center
7272 Greenville Avenue
Dallas, TX 75231-4596
1-800-242-8721
http://www.americanheart.org

Mental Health Resources

American Anorexia/Bulimia Association
165 West 46th Street, Suite 1108
New York, NY 10036
1-212-575-6200

Autism Society of American
8601 Georgia Avenue, Suite 503
Silver Spring, MD 20910
1-301-657-0881
http://www.autism-society.org

National Association of Anorexia Nervosa and Associated Disorders
PO Box 7
Highland Park, IL 60035
1-847-831-3438

National Mental Health Association
1021 Prince Street
Alexandria, VA 22314-2971
1-800-969-6642
http://www.nmha.org

Other Resources

American Burn Association
625 N. Michigan Avenue, Suite 1530
Chicago, IL 60611
1-312-642-9260

American Cleft Palate-Craniofacial Association (CPF)
104 South Estes Drive, Suite 294
Chapel Hill, NC 27514
1-919-933-9044

Cystic Fibrosis Foundation
6931 Arlington Road
Bethesda, MD 20814
1-800-FIGHTCF
http://www.cff.org

Crohn's and Colitis Foundation of America
386 Park Avenue South
17th Floor
New York, NY 10016
1-800-932-2423
http://www.ccfa.org

Epilepsy Foundation
4351 Garden City Drive
Landover, MD 20785
1-800-EFA-1000
http://www.efa.org

National Attention Deficit Disorder Association
1788 Second Street, Suite 200
Highland Park, IL 60035
1-847-432-ADDA

National Clearinghouse on Child Abuse and Neglect Information
330 C Street, SW
Washington, DC 20447
1-800-394-3366
http://www.calib.com/nccanch

National Head Injury Foundation
1776 Massachusetts Avenue, Suite 100
Washington, DC 20036
1-800-444-6443
http://www.healthy.net/pan/cso/cioi/NHIF.HTM

National Hemophilia Foundation
116 W. 32nd Street, 11th Fl.
New York, NY 10001
1-800-42-HANDI
http://www.hemophilia.org

National Organization of Rare Disorders, Inc.
Fairwood Professional Building, 100 Route 37
P.O. Box 8923
New Fairfield, CT 06812-8923
1-800-999-6673
http://www.healthy.net/pan/cso/cioi/NORD.HTM

National Pediculosis Association
PO Box 610189
Newton, MA 02161
1-800-446-4NPA
http://www.headlice.org

Neurofibromatosis Foundation
95 Pine Street, 16th Floor
New York, NY 10005
1-800-323-7938

Sickle Cell Disease Association of America
200 Corporate Point, Suite 495
Culver City, CA 90230-6363
1-800-421-8453

Sudden Infant Death Syndrome (SIDS) Alliance
1314 Bedford Avenue, Suite 210
Baltimore, MD 21208
1-410-653-8226
http://www.sidsalliance.org

REFERENCES

American Academy of Pediatrics. (2000). In L. K. Pickering (Ed.), *2000 Red book: Report of the Committee on Infectious Diseases* (25th ed.). Elk Grove Village, IL: American Academy of Pediatrics.

American Heart Association. (1997). *International Liaison Committee on Resuscitation Advisory Statements: Pediatric resuscitation* [On-line]. Available: http://216.185.112.5/presenter.jhtml?identifier=1814

Centers for Disease Control and Prevention. (1994). Revised classification system for human immunodeficiency virus infection in children less than 13 years of age. *MMWR Morbidity and Mortality Weekly Report, 43,* 1–10 (MMWR No. RR-12).

Corbett, J. V. (1996). *Laboratory tests & diagnostic procedures with nursing diagnoses* (4th ed.). Stamford, CT: Appleton & Lange.

Daniels, R. (2002). *Delmar's guide to laboratory and diagnostic tests.* Albany, NY: Delmar.

Frankenburg, W. K., & Dodds, J. B. (1990). *Denver II.* Denver: Denver Developmental Materials, Inc.

Kemper, K. J. (1997). A practical approach to chronic asthma management. *Contemporary Pediatrics, 14*(8), 86–114.

Potts, N. L., & Mandelco, B. (2002). *Pediatric nursing: Caring for children and their families.* Albany, NY: Delmar.

Rosenstein, B. J., & Fosarelli, P. D. (1997). *Pediatric pearls: The handbook of practical pediatrics* (3rd ed.). St. Louis: Mosby.

Siberry, G. K., Iannone, R., & Johns Hopkins Hospital Children's Medical and Surgical Center. (2000). *The Harriet Lane handbook: A manual for pediatric house officers—The Harriet Lane Service, Children's Medical and Surgical Center of Johns Hopkins Hospital* (15th ed.). St. Louis: Mosby.

Taketomo, C. K., Hodding, J. H., & Kraus, D. M. (1999). *Pediatric dosage handbook* (6th ed.). Cleveland: Lexi-Comp; American Pharmaceutical Association.

Wong, D. L. (2000). *Pediatric quick reference* (3rd ed.). St. Louis: Mosby.

Wong, D. L, & Whaley, L. F. (1999). *Whaley & Wong's nursing care of infants and children* (6th ed.). St. Louis: Mosby.

INDEX